JOURNEY *through* CANCER

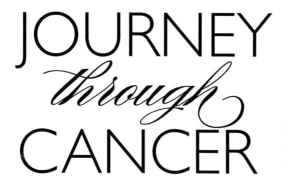

ALSO BY NEROLI DUFFY

Wanting to Be Born: The Cry of the Soul

The Practical Mystic:
Life Lessons from Conversations with Mrs. Booth

BY NEROLI DUFFY AND MARILYN BARRICK

Wanting to Live: Overcoming the Seduction of Suicide

JOURNEY *through* CANCER

A Guide to Integrating Conventional, Complementary and Spiritual Healing

DR. NEROLI DUFFY

DARJEELING PRESS
Emigrant, Montana

JOURNEY THROUGH CANCER

A Guide to Integrating Conventional, Complementary and Spiritual Healing

by Dr. Neroli Duffy

This book describes various steps that the author took in treating her cancer. There is no single formula for success, since each person's situation is different. Therefore, anyone who has cancer or who could have cancer should place himself or herself under the care of an oncologist or cancer specialist and seek professional advice before acting on any information herein. This book is sold with the understanding that no legal responsibility is assumed for the completeness or accuracy of its contents or for any actions taken by the reader in reliance on anything contained in the book. Nothing in this book is intended to diagnose, treat, prevent, or cure any disease or condition.

www.journeythroughcancer.org

To my mother, Marie Norman;

My spiritual mother and teacher, Elizabeth Clare
Prophet;

The Divine Mothers in the heaven-world,

Mother Mary of the West and Kuan Yin of the East;

and Hilarion the Healer

CONTENTS

ACKNOWLEDGEMENTS

Many thanks to:
My husband, Peter, for his love, constancy, care, and attention, for holding my hand every step of the way through the journey of healing and for holding on to the vision that healing was indeed possible;
Rev. Annice Booth, for encouraging me to write my story;
Elizabeth Clare Prophet, who taught me so many of the spiritual truths in this book;
All the embodied angels who participated in my care and through whose hands the Master of Life sent healing currents of love;
Cancer Treatment Centers of America and their staff, who give their all each day to help so many in the fight against cancer.

INTRODUCTION

It has been said that cancer is a word and not a sentence—it is the name that is given to a health challenge, not a destination. I agree with that assessment. In facing cancer I have learned to face my own fears, even my fear of death. If you are faced with cancer, one of the most important things that will determine your outcome is the kind of person that you are and how you respond. And until you face cancer, you never really know how you will respond.

Cancer has been described as a wake-up call—this was indeed true for me. I have also seen that, as hard as it is to deal with cancer, it can be a blessing in disguise.

Cancer can also be a teacher—a hard teacher, perhaps, but if you are willing to humble yourself, cancer *can* teach you profound lessons. For me, cancer was and is all of these things and more.

Cancer is also a journey. There are many different routes, and yet the path has been defined and is well-worn by the feet of those who have gone before, unwillingly perhaps, but often with courage and a fighting spirit that I have seldom seen elsewhere. The men and women I met in treatment traveled this road with me and inspired me.

The statistics say that one in four Americans at one time in their life will be faced with cancer. Breast cancer will affect one in eight women. I never expected to be one of them.

I was a forty-four-year-old medical doctor turned minister when I was diagnosed with breast cancer on January 25, 1999. I have never been one to remember dates, but this is one I have not forgotten. It was a date that was to change my life in ways that I could never imagine.

In the years since the diagnosis, I have experienced and learned so much. I can look back on the experience now and, as hard as it was, feel that I would not have changed it for the world. In many ways I feel like a different person and more of who I truly am.

This book is born out of a desire to share what I have learned throughout this growth process. It contains specific keys that not only apply to breast cancer or cancer in general but which can help anyone who desires to find healing. I especially want to share what I feel were the keys to my healing, things that I wish I had known prior to my diagnosis.

The first part of this book recounts my own experience with breast cancer—day-by-day, week-by-week. It is painful at times. Certainly, it was when I was going through it. I am sharing it here with the hope that others may learn from it, as I learned so much from the experience of many others who faced cancer.

In the second part of this book, I have distilled what I have learned about cancer and its treatment into some practical guidelines that others who are facing cancer can use in their own healing journey. I happened to have breast cancer, but the principles I applied can be used for any kind of cancer.

In the third part of the book, I explore and expand on the subject of cancer as a spiritual teacher and illness as a spiritual journey.

Above all, I learned that cancer is not just a disease of a particular organ. It affects the whole person, and it responds best to an approach that treats the whole person. If you approach the challenge of cancer in this way, you may find that the journey through cancer becomes a journey toward healing at all levels of body, mind, and spirit.

I have chosen to call this book *Journey through Cancer* because for me it has truly been a personal journey in healing. I also hope it can provide some guideposts for your personal healing journey, whatever it might be. In one sense, the healing journey never ends. Healing and wholeness are things we seek throughout our lives, be they at physical, emotional, or spiritual levels.

My experience with breast cancer was a key turning point in my own healing journey. I had a burning desire to document the journey, and the journaling of my experience was also a means to help me through my own healing process. I worked on the book as I traveled down that uncertain road that has been called the "cancer experience."

But before I share the techniques that helped me, I would like to share with you a little bit about myself—who I am and what I find important in life.

IF YOU ARE FACED WITH CANCER, ONE OF THE MOST IMPORTANT THINGS THAT WILL DETERMINE YOUR OUTCOME IS THE KIND OF PERSON YOU ARE AND HOW YOU RESPOND.

PROLOGUE

I have long known that there are many reasons for diseases to manifest in the body—the visible symptoms are simply the final result of a cause-effect sequence that begins a long time before the illness manifests itself physically. My own internal compass, my studies, and later, my own life and my experience with patients and their illnesses taught me this. These beliefs are not new for me, but grew naturally out of my experiences early in life.

I was born in Perth, Western Australia, in 1954. My father and mother were self-confessed spiritual seekers, always searching for Truth, and I, along with two brothers and a sister, was raised almost from birth with the understanding that life is a spiritual journey and earth a schoolroom. In our family, the universe was a place in which to learn the lessons of life, and this physical world was but a shadow of the real world that existed just beyond the veil. I believed in angels and beings of light who guide and protect us, and as a child I felt their comforting presence about me.

My parents did not have to tell me about angels. I have always believed in them, ever since I saw one at the foot of my bed as a little girl. I don't see angels now, but I know that they are real, I work with them daily and I often feel them working in my life. I especially felt their presence when I developed breast cancer.

My parents also taught me that there is truth in all the world's major religions. They explained that there are good people in all walks of life who are on their way to heaven; they are merely taking different routes up the mountain. I was taught that no one form of devotion is better than another and that one should respect them all.

My parents explained the concepts of karma and reincarnation in ways that a child could understand, and I began to see these principles at work in my family and in my life. I also observed how energy affects each of us and how what we send out, good or ill, comes back to us like a boomerang. I knew that I had lived before and that I would live again when I laid this body down at the end of this earthly life. I learned from an early age that my past affects the present even as I build my future by the choices I make each day.

Our family discussed the mysteries of life around the dinner table every evening. And often, long after the meal was over, our talk lingered late into the night. Eventually, Dad got up and washed the dishes, we four children dried them, and my mother put them back in the cupboards, all the while continuing our conversations.

The kitchen was the gathering place in our home, and although we did not have abundant material wealth, we were rich in love and spiritual blessings. Back then, we had an old wood stove that we used for cooking and warming the house. I loved to come home and smell the aroma of fresh-baked bread and beautiful home-cooked meals that emerged from that old black oven. We all gathered in the kitchen after school and work to talk about our day and share the love of family.

As a child and a teenager, I had an intense desire to learn more about healing—in the spiritual as well as the physical sense. My parents taught me that there is more to a human being than what we see. I learned that we are all spiritual beings who happen to occupy physical bodies. I soon became aware of the connection between my body and my mind and saw how my emotions affected my body.

For many years I worked with my Higher Self, whom I think of as my chief guardian angel, and I continue to do so today. I believe that we can all call upon the assistance of our inner guides if we learn to listen to that gentle voice speaking within us. This was to be one of the great lessons that I learned anew with cancer as my teacher.

I grew up with all of these wondrous concepts, and I became a medical doctor out of a desire to help, serve, and heal others. But in the 1960s, when I was growing up, and even in the 1970s, when I was a medical student and later an intern, these were unusual subjects for much of the world, and especially the medical community.

And so, when I was in medical school, I kept these things to myself. At home, at night, I was encouraged to "keep an open mind" to spiritual subjects. But at medical school during the day, I desperately wanted to fit in with my friends and fellow students. For indeed, I often felt "different" and "strange." At the time, I wondered if our family was strange too. What if we were the only family who thought like this?

I remember coming home one night and asking my father if there were others in the world with whom I could talk about these subjects. He, in his wisdom, smiled and said, "Yes, there are many others in the world who are searching for truth and who have open minds. And one day, later in life, you will find them." At the time I trusted his words, and yet I wondered how he could possibly know. Now I know that he was right, and I have found these seekers everywhere and in all walks of life.

I began medical school with such high hopes but soon learned that there is a big difference between medicine and healing. I knew, for example, that we had finer spiritual bodies beyond the physical flesh that we wear, which doctors treat. I felt that there were so many other avenues for healing besides writing a prescription, but we were not encouraged to talk about them. When I broached these subjects I quickly found that the medical community was not receptive. So I learned to keep silent.

I did very well in my studies and was one of the finalists in the prize for medicine in my final year exams. I particularly enjoyed the study of psychology and won the prize for this subject. Like many in my class, I was a good student and a hard-working doctor. I took delight in the details of the diagnostic process, seeing how it all came together to reveal the problem and to find the solution for each individual patient.

I loved to talk with people, and I was always interested in the person behind the patient. We were taught that a careful and detailed medical history could reveal much and that 90 percent of the medical diagnosis was made on the history that the patient gave or that the doctor elicited from the patient. Yet surprisingly few doctors took the time to really listen to their patients or even to ask the right questions.

It seemed natural to me that if you talked with the patient, they usually told you what the problem was—not always in so many words but often in unmistakable ways. One example I clearly remember is a patient who had suffered a severe head trauma. He had no family to care for him, and he came into the hospital for investigation in order to decide what he would be permitted to do. Was he able to drive a car, care for himself, and so forth?

Some of the doctors thought that he was functioning normally. As a final-year medical student, I spent over an hour with him and noticed the subtle signs of injury to the brain. In medical terms, I found him to be *disinhibited*—he lacked the normal boundaries that one would expect in conversation and behavior. There was also a bluntness in the way he spoke and a lack of spontaneity. All of this revealed the subtle effects of an injury to the frontal lobe—the area of the brain that influences personality. To me, it was simply evident in who he was, what he was saying, and how he was saying it, and the specialist neurologist agreed. I do not think that I was more intelligent than the others who had not seen the problem, but I had taken the time to talk to the patient, to listen and to observe.

I graduated from the University of Western Australia Medical School in 1979 after six years of intense study and an additional year of research, earning a Bachelor of Medical Science with First Class Honors. I decided to intern at Royal Perth Hospital, a teaching hospital where I had received a large part of my training as a medical student. I saw myself eventually working in a country town somewhere in Australia, so I worked to broaden my medical horizons and get the experience that I would need to practice rural medicine, where specialists are many hours away and a single doctor may have to deal with every kind of medical problem.

Besides the usual medical and surgical internships that a new doctor is required to do, I did rotations in plastic surgery, orthopedics, neurosurgery, oncology, psychiatry, neurology, geriatrics, intensive care, and emergency care. In my second year I was stationed for a time in Kalgoorlie, a mining town in the desert of Western Australia. I later worked for six months each in pediatrics, obstetrics, and gynecology, because my professors had told me that as a female doctor in rural practice, I would be inundated with women and children.

After three years of internship, I joined the Family Medical Program run by the Royal Australian College of General Practitioners, which gave me the opportunity to work in the outback of Western Australia. I also had the opportunity to fly with the Royal Flying Doctor Service, stationed at Derby, a very small town in the remote northwest corner of Australia. Several times a week, I would fly, along with a nurse, a pilot, and often another doctor, into some even more remote settlement to set up a clinic for the day.

Life as a doctor was very busy and involved a lot of hard work. I loved it in many ways, even though it left me little time for a life of my own. My last hospital job was as a registrar in anesthesia, including rotations in intensive care and emergency. I spent a total of two and a half years in anesthesia, including a year in England earning a Diploma of Anesthesia from the Royal College of Surgeons in London. I loved anesthesia and at one time seriously considered it for my life's profession. However, the universe had other plans for me.

I learned a lot about life during my time as a registrar in anesthesia. Each week, I was assigned a list of patients scheduled for surgery. One aspect of my job was to visit the patients the night before their surgery, take their history, examine them, answer any questions they might have, allay their concerns, and prescribe preoperative medication. The next

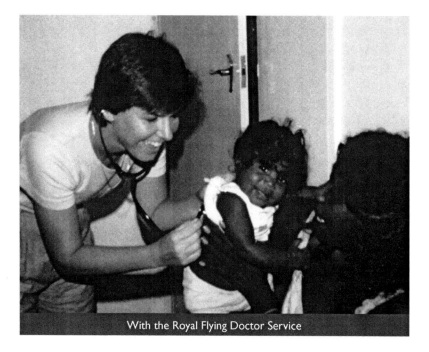

With the Royal Flying Doctor Service

morning I would anesthetize them for their surgery. The preoperative visit was the main point of conscious patient contact, and even though it might appear to be routine, it was actually a very important part of anesthesia, as an anxious patient is more difficult to put to sleep.

I enjoyed these preoperative visits. I became aware that the patients liked to know who was putting them to sleep and to meet the person who would be caring for them while they were in surgery. I loved being a part of the team that worked in the operating room, working alongside the surgeons and nurses. I loved the order and cleanliness of the operating room, and I felt great satisfaction when the anesthesia went smoothly.

My only sadness was that I really did not get to spend a lot of time with the patients. They were asleep during their surgery, and by the time they woke up fully, they were back in their bed on the ward. I would sometimes visit them after the procedure, but often there was no time, since I was already on to the next case. Outpatients simply went home, and I did not see them again.

I saw medicine as a science, but also an art. And my own emerging spiritual life was teaching me about the more subtle aspects of that art. I was beginning to note the influence of the emotions and the mind on patients and how this was reflected in their illnesses. How I longed then for books on the deeper meaning of illness and the effects of more subtle forms of energy and modes of healing.

Later, I quietly began to use spiritual tools such as prayer in my medical practice and noticed amazing results. At times I was very aware of a guiding presence helping me. I used to think of it as an angel sitting on my shoulder, whispering in my ear, telling me what to look for or what test to perform. Of course, I followed medical guidelines and procedures, but I was also open to what my angels or my Higher Self had to say. I never told my fellow doctors or nurses or even my patients that I prayed for them. But I clearly observed the effects of prayer in faster healing, changes in lifestyle, greater comfort and increased awareness of the meaning of illness. One example out of many comes to mind.

One middle-aged woman was recovering from cancer of the bladder. She needed a brief anesthetic every three months for a cystoscopy, a short procedure in which a specialist inspected the bladder for signs of recurrence of the cancer. Although the procedure itself was quick and patients would normally go home within a few hours, this woman often required admission to the hospital due to the effects of the anesthetic. This had been a pattern for her for several years. Every three months she underwent the cystoscopy and then had to stay in the hospital for up to three days to recover.

When I went to see her for the preoperative visit, I could see that she was very concerned, and understandably so. She had been anesthetized many times by many specialists using different techniques, but the results were always the same—nausea and vomiting for three days. On reviewing her medical notes, it became clear that every possible method for dealing with her problem had been tried before. I had nothing new to offer medically—but I did tell her that I would try something new.

That night, and again the next day when she was asleep on the operating table, I prayed for her and asked that her soul be taken to temples of light in the heaven-world. I also whispered in her ear once she was asleep that she would wake up without any symptoms. She would be very comfortable. She would not have any nausea, nor would she be in pain. (This was in the days before I knew about the work of such pioneers in the field of mind-body medicine as Dr. Bernie Siegel.)

It worked extremely well. When I went to visit her, she was sitting up in bed, beaming from ear to ear. She asked me what I had done. She had no side effects whatsoever and was ready to go home, a first! I told her that it was really no secret—I had simply prayed for her. I told her what to ask for in her prayers and I said that she could do the same for herself the next time she needed to have a cystoscopy. Years later, I was to use the same techniques on myself when I underwent surgery for breast cancer.

As much as I loved anesthesia, I did not feel it was the way I wanted to spend the rest of my days. In 1985, I made an abrupt change and returned to family medicine. My final years as a doctor were spent seeing patients in the new Perth suburb of Mirrabooka, in a medical practice with five other doctors. My waiting room was always full, and I often ran late: if someone needed to talk or take longer for their consultation, I rarely refused. Most of the patients who were waiting knew that I would do the same for them and did not seem to mind the wait.

I practiced anesthesia and family medicine for ten years. As I look back now, I realize that I loved medicine but I often felt drained and unhappy. I fully understood the great benefits of surgery and anesthesia and the life-saving effects of many medical procedures and modern medications. These are surely gifts that have been given to us that have brought us out of the dark ages. However, at the same time, I was dissatisfied with the limitations of traditional medicine and knew in my heart that there had to be a higher way. I felt that the subtle dimensions of illness, particularly the mind-body connection and certain alternative forms of treatment, were not being accorded the attention they deserved.

How I wished I had known people like Bernie Siegel, Christiane Northrup, or Joan Borysenko, who have written so eloquently on alternative approaches to medicine. I would not have felt so alone among my peers. There was a whole other side of myself that I often simply had to keep hidden. Only my family and a few fellow seekers of truth and spirituality understood.

And then, in 1989, my life took an even more abrupt turn as I left the medical field to join the ministry. That is a story in itself. Ten years earlier I would have said that it was unthinkable that I would leave medicine. I had felt called to medicine and had worked hard to become a doctor. And yet, this was another calling.

I had joined The Summit Lighthouse, a spiritual organization, some years earlier and found in its teachings many of the answers my soul had been seeking. I met my future husband, Peter, a fellow Australian living in America. After we married and I moved to America, I became a minister in Church Universal and Triumphant, the church affiliated with The Summit Lighthouse. We now live and work in Paradise Valley in the mountains of southwest Montana.

Although I no longer practice medicine, I came to see that I had not really left the healing profession. I simply moved on to a different and more subtle kind of healing—the healing of the soul, the spirit, and the finer bodies. I teach at Summit University, the educational arm of The Summit Lighthouse, where I lecture on a diverse range of topics, including spiritual healing. I have lost neither my love for medicine and healing nor my love and appreciation for the people who work in those fields. As a doctor and a minister I have found a new freedom to discuss medicine and healing within the framework of the spiritual journey.

As I look back on my transition from medicine to ministry, I see there were many clues as to the direction my life would take. I can still vividly recall the last days of my medical practice in Western Australia. By this time my younger sister, Margo, had graduated as a doctor and joined the practice. And those professors were right! Margo and I were inundated with women and their children seeking to be treated and cared for by other women.

Many wonderful and special things happened, and I treasure those times with our patients, but for some reason one particular patient has stayed in my mind for many years. She was one of the last patients I treated before I left, and she happened to be a patient with breast cancer.

Cheryl was about forty years of age when she first came into my office. I spent many hours with her and witnessed her suffering firsthand. I was with her in her final hours as she was cared for at home by her loving mother and hospice nurses. She died after a long and valiant fight, and witnessing the course of her illness had a profound effect on me.

When I was diagnosed with breast cancer in 1999, I remembered Cheryl. Only this time I was not a spectator or assistant at the bedside. This time it was *me* who was going through the experience of cancer. Somehow it was easy to see myself walking that same path—a long and painful illness ending in death. I thought of the phrase in the Bible, "Physician, heal thyself,"[1] and I knew that this would be a test of all that I had learned of healing and medicine and of all that I had learned of the spiritual path.

I returned to study and sought to discover all that I could about cancer, illness, and healing—with a renewed interest and a new impetus, prompted by the need to survive. This time, I was the patient and not the doctor.

I had understood from childhood that there are no accidents in life, that everything happens for a reason, even if we cannot always see it at the time. We have all come to earth for a higher purpose, and I believed and trusted in a Higher Power and a life plan that was more vast and beautiful than we could possibly imagine. Cancer helped me to understand more and more my place in that plan, and I believed that for me, whether I lived or died as a result of having cancer, it could be another forward step in that plan.

We are all unique in what we bring to the experience of healing and the choices we might make. Nevertheless, I learned much from those who went before me in this journey—those who wrote about their experiences and those I met along the way who shared their stories with me. I also learned that while our experiences were unique, we had much in common.

I believe that healing is truly a journey, a pilgrimage that is different for each one. For all of us, this journey takes time and there are steps to take and places to visit along the way—and many of those places we all visit at one time or another.

So before I share my road map for navigating through this unfamiliar land, I will share my story. I don't consider my experience to be either typical or exceptional. It is simply another story of the journey. I share it in the hope that you might find something helpful for your own journey—to realize that while no one can walk it for you, others have gone before, and you need never walk it alone.

A journey in healing is what this book is all about—and all journeys begin with that first step.

SECTION I

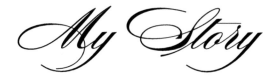

My Story

Chapter 1

THIS WASN'T SUPPOSED TO HAPPEN TO ME

I had always done regular breast exams. After all, I was a doctor, and I knew the importance of breast self-examination. When I was thirty-six years old, a year after I married, I developed a large, painful lump in the right breast just prior to my monthly cycle. I was used to small lumpy areas that would come and go with the menstrual cycle, but this one really worried me. It seemed to develop quite quickly and was about two to three centimeters wide and quite tender. I saw a surgeon, and he felt that it was related to the hormone fluctuations of my monthly cycles, but he was prepared to do a biopsy if it did not disappear. He reviewed it again in a week and it had totally disappeared, proving that it was related to the menstrual cycle. I was greatly relieved. I had been worried that it might be cancer or have cancer underlying it.

I continued my breast exams monthly and did not notice any problems. Then, for several months towards the end of 1998, I noticed a thickening in my right breast in the upper-outer quadrant. At the time, I was not worried about it and didn't think that it could be anything serious. Furthermore, it did not feel like a lump to me. I thought about it now and then, but I mostly forgot about the fact that it was there. I never even called it a "lump." This seems very odd when I think back on it now. Why would I, as a doctor, not recognize a lump for what it was.

Around the same time, I remarked to my secretary that I really needed to have a mammogram. (This was not prompted by the breast "thickening," or at least not consciously—I never made this connection at the time.) I was forty-four years old and had never had a mammogram and had thought that by my forty-fifth birthday I would begin to have them regularly. I would remember the mammogram from time to time, and I made an appointment in November to have one, as well as a Pap smear, routine blood work, and an annual checkup. I was not able to attend on the appointed day because of my busy work schedule, so I made a mental note to book again in the new year.

In the meantime, my husband, Peter, and I flew back to Australia for Christmas. It was the first Christmas we had spent with his family since our marriage ten years earlier. I was lying in bed on the morning of New Year's Day thinking about nothing in particular, when my hand went to my breast and I felt the area again. This time it seemed more pronounced and "thicker." In my own mind, even then, I did not call it a lump or even think of it as a lump. I told Peter about it and we agreed that I would get it checked when I got back to Montana. I did not tell anyone else, certainly not my family members, who were enjoying the holiday season.

My medical training had taught me that any breast lump was cancer until proven otherwise, and I had always urged women to get breast lumps properly assessed. In my medical practice I had never adopted a wait-and-see attitude with breast lumps. If a friend or a patient had come to me with the same symptoms I would have gone with them to get a mammogram that day. But somehow, even though I was uneasy, I never really thought that it could be cancer. Near the end of my treatment, I came to realize that I had been in denial and had simply not wanted to consider the possibility. I guess that's why you cannot be your own doctor.

So on Monday, January 25, 1999, I drove to a clinic in Montana to see the gynecologist for a Pap smear and checkup, followed by what was supposed to be a routine mammogram. In the course of the examination, she checked my breasts. She noticed the lump and questioned me about it. She was clearly concerned and wanted me to have the mammogram right away. She stopped talking gynecology and focused on the lump. She called it a lump. She said, "Breast lumps are always distressing things to find, and it's always an uneasy time until you find out what is happening." She seemed to be thinking that there was a strong possibility of this "lump" being cancer. "No way! She is wrong! This is not cancer," is what was going through my mind. And yet, I was relieved. I had wanted the mammogram.

So off I went to have the mammogram at the local hospital. After the mammogram, the technician came back in the room for "more views of the right breast." Then the radiologist came in and said that they wanted to do an ultrasound. Fine. I was feeling calm when I went to the ultrasound room. The radiologist and technician were chatting amiably with me until they began to focus on the lump. I heard them say that it was solid and not cystic (fluid filled). They measured it to be two centimeters in diameter. Their routine chatter stopped and they looked at me and explained what was going on.

By this time I felt that I was in someone else's bad dream. I switched to my familiar doctor mode and I said to myself, "I have no risk factors for breast cancer except that I have not had children. A solid lump in a woman aged forty-four with no children and no risk factors means that cancer is on the list of possibilities. Two centimeters means if it is cancer, it is probably at least stage II.* It could also have spread to the lymph system, or microscopically into the blood, which would make it

---

* Breast cancer is categorized as stage I – IV, depending on the size of the lump and whether it has spread to other tissues. Stage I is a lump of less than two centimeters with no evidence of cancer in the lymph nodes or elsewhere in the body. The probability of a good outcome is much higher if breast cancer is detected at this early stage.

stage III or IV."

Images of Cheryl, my breast-cancer patient who died, were running through my mind. But this was not Australia, and I was not Cheryl. This was America, this was me, and this was definitely not supposed to be happening. And yet, I knew how this scene plays out. I had been there before. Only now I was the one on the table in the thin, short gown, with the white cotton blanket over me, feeling suddenly cold and hot at the same time.

The radiologist was very kind. He said all the right things—all the things that my training had taught me to say. They could not tell what it was without a biopsy. And yet it seemed to be written all over his face what he really thought: "Nice young woman, forty-four years old, with right-sided breast cancer, probably at least stage II. What a shame." I felt as if I could read his mind. He and the technicians were worried for me. I could read the concern on their faces. And that was when I knew that I had breast cancer. I just knew.

From that point on, everything was blurry and out of focus. It felt like my life was on fast forward and slow motion, frame by frame, at the same time. The hospital staff were very kind, and I knew their concern was genuine. Their kindness melted all my self-control. My medical reserve was gone and I was now a patient. I began to cry.

They said and did everything in the best possible way and with compassion, and it was right for them not to tell me what they thought. After all, you never know. It might not be cancer, and you have to wait for the results of the biopsy, no matter what you think. But I was no longer a statistic or a probability. This was me! Tears tumbled down my cheeks as I lay on the X-ray table and they searched for a surgeon to see me right away. *This was not supposed to be happening to me.*

I got up and got dressed and called Peter on the phone in the little change room. I cried again and asked him to make the fifty-mile drive to the hospital. Before Peter could get there, the surgeon came to see me. He had been just a few feet away in the operating room of this small country hospital. He very kindly came out between cases, still wearing his light-blue surgical gear. He was young with a little gray hair at the temples. His touch and manner were gentle, and he seemed genuinely concerned. I remember that his hands were warm. I had often noticed that good surgeons tend to have what I would call "surgeon's hands"— strong, clean from years of scrubbing up, warm to the touch. This man had the hands of a surgeon, and my years of working with surgeons told me that he was a capable one.

He talked to me and then examined me. He knew my medical background. I asked him what he thought of the lump. He acknowledged the possibility that it might be cancer. He declined to say what he thought, preferring to see what the biopsy showed. I did not really expect him to answer that question, but somehow I had to ask. But again, I knew from his face.

We talked about what would happen if the biopsy was positive. He said he would have to sample some lymph nodes to determine what stage it was. My breasts were small and he was not sure that he could get a good cosmetic result with lumpectomy. He seemed to be leaning towards mastectomy. That scared me. For a while, the doctor in me took over. I asked him all of my questions, and he very patiently answered them all. He talked of several "worrisome" additional areas of calcification on the mammogram in another quadrant of the same breast that would need to be checked. He was concerned about multi-focal disease. I said that I was not opposed to mastectomy if that was required, but I wanted to be sure about my options. He agreed and said that we could go step by step.

During the course of the half-hour consultation, we talked about all aspects of treatment. I asked a lot of questions, almost on autopilot from my medical days. I asked about lymph-node dissection, simple versus radical mastectomy, chemotherapy, radiation, estrogen-receptor status, needle biopsy versus biopsy. Part of me could not believe that I was talking about these things. Within such a short space of time, my life had begun to feel unreal, and I felt that I had just lost control. I remember thinking, "This is how it feels to be told that you have cancer."

Why me?

Well, why not me? Had I thought that I was special and somehow protected and that it could not happen to me?

I wondered at how quickly things can change in your life. In the space of half an hour, I was talking to a surgeon about losing my breast and possibly undergoing chemotherapy.

I really, really wanted to know whether or not it was cancer. And I wanted to know *now*. I asked if he could do the biopsy that same day—perhaps hoping that somehow, it wasn't really cancer. His busy schedule did not allow it—and probably just as well. It might have been too much for one day. We scheduled for three days later. The surgeon left for his next case. I got changed and met Peter, who had just arrived in the hospital corridor. He was great, calm as always and practical, loving, and very supportive. I loved him so much in that moment.

We hugged and talked. Let's take it one step at a time. Maybe the biopsy will be negative. If it is positive, maybe it will be early-stage. Let's look at all the options.

That night, Peter felt the lump himself and said, "Yes, it really is a lump. It is quite noticeable, isn't it?" I felt a little foolish and un-doctor-like. Peter could feel it easily once it had been pointed out to him. Yes, there was no mistaking that it was a lump, although I had not really called it that before.

This "lump" now occupied my waking and sleeping hours. The concerns of my job and all those things that had seemed so important now faded into the background as the issue of life and death loomed before me. I went back to work for part of each day, almost mechanically, and although I functioned pretty well, not all of me was there. A lot of me was ten years in the past, with Cheryl, reliving her life and wondering if that was indeed the path before me. I felt as if it was.

I knew the power of prayer, so I called my coworkers and friends to ask them to pray for me. I was not reticent about telling them what was going on with my life, and I welcomed their support. One church member, a single mother with small children whose husband had died of cancer some years before, had recently been through a similar experience. She had discovered a breast lump and was scheduled for further tests. She had prayed and the lump disappeared. I called and asked her to pray for me.

As a member of the board of directors of our organization, I attended a board meeting the night before surgery, and everyone wished me well. They assured me that surely all would be well. I felt that way too. Surely all will be well. Part of me believed in miracles. Part of me held onto the possibility that it would not be breast cancer. However, another part of me felt sure that I had cancer. I kept thinking of Cheryl and other breast-cancer patients that I had known. Somehow, I could only think of the ones who were no longer with us.

In the early afternoon of Thursday, January 28, I went back to the hospital with Peter and had the breast biopsy. It was done under local anesthetic and they allowed Peter to be with me during the operation. The surgeon was assisted by a lovely scrub nurse who kept me busy with small talk and made sure that Peter was doing okay. It was great to have him with me. It felt weird to be operated on, literally "under my nose," and it felt strange for the surgeon to be pulling and tugging and digging around in my right breast. It did not hurt much at all—only the sting as the local anesthetic went in.

I was trying to be a model patient. I tend to be a caregiver, looking out for others, even at my own expense. I was calm and talking to everyone. I could tell from the phone calls that the surgeon had other serious cases on his schedule, and I knew what it felt like to be busy and to have patients waiting. I had heard him talking about a man with a bowel obstruction who needed surgery very soon, and he had arranged the operating room for that afternoon. I remember expressing my concern for him and thanking him for fitting me into his busy schedule that day.

The surgeon removed the entire lump, and I was left with a three-centimeter scar on my breast. I looked down and was pleased that he had done a subcuticular stitch, meaning the suture material was under the skin and that the scar would be less obvious. I told him that it was a good job and that I was grateful.

I got the impression that normally I would have had to wait several days for the result. But he knew I wanted to know, and I had asked about a frozen section of the lump (meaning a pathologist could take a preliminary look at the tissue under a microscope that day). So they sent the lump by taxi to a pathologist in a larger hospital thirty minutes away. Peter and I went to do a little shopping while all this was taking place. Two hours later, the surgeon told me that the result was "positive."

For a few seconds I thought that "positive" was good. Then I realized what "positive" meant—positive for cancer. For the first time, I was struck by the irony that we use the word "positive" in such a way.

I was not surprised that it was cancer, and yet there was a part of me that was still hoping for a different outcome. I said to him, "You were pretty sure that it would be cancer, weren't you?"

He said, "Yes. But you never know for sure."

I told him that although I knew that he couldn't say it, I had sensed his feeling when he first spoke to me.

I know how the sixth sense works in medicine. I recall many an occasion when a patient would walk into my office, and upon first hearing their symptoms, sometimes before they even said anything, I just knew what the problem was. There are physical clues—the way that a patient holds himself or the physical signs of his illness—and doctors tend to look for these signs and note them. However, there is a more subtle sense that many doctors develop with years of experience. It is a part of the art of medicine. It is as if the illness emits an aura and announces itself. All illnesses have a calling card.

We talked about my options. He was not sure that he had gotten it all and would have to wait for the pathology. He would have to sample the lymph nodes. This would be done at the same time as a mastectomy or in a separate operation. He was still concerned about the additional areas of calcification that the radiologist had called "worrisome." He would prefer to deal with it all by performing a mastectomy. He was prepared to perform the surgery the following Monday.

I asked him what he would recommend if I were his wife. He said without hesitation, "Mastectomy." I said that I wanted a second opinion, and he gave me the names of several surgeons in a larger city. He recommended one who had disagreed with him in the past in order to give me a chance to get an opinion that might not match his. I appreciated his honesty and openness.

I had been around surgeons a lot and I felt that he was good at his job, and I was grateful that such a good surgeon was there when I needed him. I told him that if I did decide on a mastectomy, I would return to him for the surgery, as I liked him and trusted him. I meant it. He treated me very kindly and took time to explain everything. I made an appointment to see him early the next week to review the final pathology.

Peter and I left the clinic, and I thought I was holding up pretty well. I felt quite calm. Then the surgical nurse came out to the car as we were pulling away and asked me how things had turned out. She had not heard from the doctor and wanted to know the biopsy result. She was very kind when I told her that it was cancer, that the surgeon recommended mastectomy, and that I was getting a second opinion. Then I started to cry. I was beginning to cry when people were nice to me.

As Peter drove us home, I used my cell phone to call the various friends and family members who had been praying for me. They were waiting to hear what was happening and I felt an urgency to let them know. I was pretty upbeat. I think that they thought I was doing "really well." I thought that I was too. But looking back, the reality of the situation had not hit me yet.

However, life was anything but the same. Suddenly, through the lens of cancer, everything else in life was becoming very clear and focused. I knew that this is what happens to people who are undergoing a sudden change in their life. I had also seen it in my patients and in my ministerial practice over and over, and here I was, observing it firsthand.

It was now easy to see what was important and what was not. Things that I had thought were crucial simply faded into the background. One thing in particular became very clear from the time that the surgeon told me that I had breast cancer: very quickly and clearly I heard a quiet voice inside my head say, "You do not have to go to work now. You have a very good excuse." I also noticed that I was very happy about that. In fact, I was almost euphoric. Was it almost worth it to get cancer so I could get out of work? I knew that this, in itself, was a very big problem, something I would have to work on at all levels.

As I looked back, I realized that I had thought about leaving almost weekly over the previous six months. I was no longer enjoying my work; in fact, I was feeling hopelessly trapped. Unable to stay but unable to leave, I somehow just kept going. I locked away my feelings, no longer looking at them or even acknowledging them. In a humorous way, I had begun to think, "This job is killing me." I had even said this to Peter and a few close friends. My secretary reminded me that I had said this to her several times.

All of this was to become very significant in my journey through cancer, and finding resolution to these issues was to be an important part of my healing experience. I did return to work for the same organization eight months later, but it was after I had completed my healing journey, and it was under very different circumstances. By that time, I was also a different person.

The next Sunday morning, Peter and I went to church. Elizabeth Clare Prophet, my spiritual teacher and the leader of our church, came and sat with us. She had called me as soon as she heard, and I was very touched by her prayers for me. Her words of comfort and concern were a great support. In church that day, she sat between us, holding our hands during the entire service. She told us to put our prayer books down so that we could hold her hands, as this was more important. I could tell that she was sending me light and healing energy for the ordeal ahead. As the service ended, I knelt at the altar rail and the tears streamed down my face. Somehow, her holding my hand had made the cancer a reality. That was the moment when it really hit me that I had cancer and that I could die. She had given me two precious gifts: the ability to see the reality of my situation and the strength to face what I had not been able to face before.

That afternoon, I could not stop crying. I thought a lot about Cheryl. I recalled every detail of her surgery, her illness, and its treatment. I remember her fading away before my eyes. I prayed and could find little comfort, feeling that I was going to die. I talked to Peter. I talked to a very dear friend who was also a minister. I told her what was on my heart and shared my fears and she listened. I was thinking that it was my time to die and feeling as if it was already happening. And I was very, very scared. Even though I had strong faith and spirituality, I was no longer a minister or a doctor. I was just another patient with some very big decisions to make.

I had begun to keep a journal. It was comforting to express myself on paper, and it enabled the thoughts to clarify and emotions to flow. Here are some of the notes that I took at the time.

Journal Entry
February 1, 1999

I stayed home from work and looked after myself. I had a whole plan of action for what to do in order to nurture and support myself. I was almost euphoric for the whole day that I would not be going to work, and I knew that was a serious sign. Was this the only way out?

At first, I was very calm. Margo [my sister] and Peter both had good feelings about the outcome. When people were sympathetic with me I cried, but not very much—just a few tears, and then I was strong again. I cried a little bit when the nurse came out to the car and asked me for the result. I called a bunch of people. Everyone was tremendously supportive and many people are praying. My sister called radiologists, surgeons and oncologists in Australia. Peter got on the Internet and printed out about two inches of information on cancer.

I prayed and I stopped working. I was mostly relieved not to have to go to work. I had been feeling the need for balance and exercise and better diet and less stress. I can no longer live in such an environment. I know that if God allows me to live, I will go on with the ministry work, but I will not go back to the job that I had. I feel that I am done with it. In a funny way, I feel that I was rescued. One night I dreamt about giving birth to a little boy called Daniel. The next night, I dreamed of a little girl. But this is not possible just now.

At first, I did not care whether I lived or died. A friend said to me, "You are a doctor. Couldn't you see it coming?" I told her that I could see it now, I guess, but I could not see it then. She said that it has devastated her and that she does not know what she can do to help me. I asked her to pray.

Later that afternoon, I did not feel like eating, and Peter and I went for a walk. I felt that I was going to die. An ice-cold grip of fear grabbed my soul and my heart. I felt the blood run from my face and I broke out in a cold sweat. I could feel a dark depression sweeping over me in a tidal wave of sadness and fear of impending death. I remembered many things, including Cheryl and her long and painful death from breast cancer. It was a terrible time.

For a little while I was beside myself, and I called a dear friend. She listened and prayed with me. I felt that I had been there before. She said that I could call her any time, day or night. Several others said the same, and it was a great reassurance to know that they were there. That night I felt the need to laugh, so Peter and I watched the movie The Wedding Singer. *It was very funny and I laughed so much. It felt good to laugh. Talk about a yo-yo—I am up one minute and down the next.*

Early this morning I got up to go to the bathroom, and when I got back to bed again, pain and fear gripped me, and my chest ached. I felt alone in the dark and that I was dying. Peter woke up and talked to me and held me for half an hour before the alarm went off. It was such a comfort. He listened to me and even made me laugh once or twice.

When he went to work I sat up in bed, said a rosary of surrender, and gave it all to God and to Mother Mary. I felt a sense of peace and comfort and found that it really helped me a lot. I made an appointment with a counselor today. She managed to fit me into her schedule, and seeing her provided great support. We talked of many things—the dark night of the soul, my fear of death, and the feeling that I am dying. I made another appointment to see her, and I feel that things are lifting. She said that the funny videos are a great idea, and that I may find myself crying also. It is okay to cry, and I need to grieve.

Somehow it helps if I write lists. Here is what I have been doing since I found out about the diagnosis:

1. *Loving myself more and not being so hard on myself*
2. *Meditating and visualizing*
3. *Applying the remedy recommended by Edgar Cayce: castor-oil packs to the breasts*
4. *Sleeping a lot*

5. *Taking vitamins and supplements to boost my immune system and St. John's Wort for depression*

6. *Reading about Padre Pio, the Catholic saint. I like him because he says, "Pray, hope, and don't worry."*

7. *Attending therapy sessions*

8. *Looking at my thoughts and changing the way that I think*

9. *Talking to Peter a lot and giving him a lot of love—and loving myself*

10. *Reading and studying about breast cancer*

TIPS FOR THE NEWLY DIAGNOSED

- "This is not supposed to be happening to me!" is a common reaction.
- Don't be surprised if you find yourself on an emotional roller coaster.
- Seek spiritual support and ask people to pray for you.
- Don't be weighed down by the recall of someone else's journey.
- Hang onto hope—no matter how small it might seem at first, it can grow.
- Allow others to help you.
- Keeping a journal can be surprisingly useful—expressing yourself on paper is comforting and enables thoughts to clarify and emotions to flow.

CHAPTER 2

MY EXPERIENCE WITH BREAST-CANCER PATIENTS

A s I faced my own diagnosis, I thought back to the many patients I had seen over the years who had been in this situation.

After becoming a doctor, I worked for a time as a resident in oncology, radiotherapy, surgery, and plastic surgery and had seen many breast-cancer patients. In the several years I worked in anesthesia, I anesthetized a number of patients for breast surgery. In those times, radical mastectomy was a common treatment for breast cancer. In this operation (virtually never performed these days), the whole breast is removed along with all of the lymph nodes under the arm up as far as the collarbone and the muscles going from the chest to the shoulder (pectoralis major and pectoralis minor). It is a disfiguring operation and often results in lymphedema or permanent limitation in the use of the arm.*

---

* The "total mastectomy" that is performed these days involves removal of the breast but not the muscles under the breast tissue, so movement of the arm is usually not affected severely. Fewer lymph nodes are removed, so lymphedema is less likely. (Lymphedema is swelling of the arm caused by accumulation of fluid that would normally be drained by the lymph nodes in the armpit.)

Later, in my family medical practice, I saw many women—as a woman doctor, they just seemed to gravitate towards me. Some of them had breast cancer. I discovered breast lumps on routine examinations. I examined breast lumps after women discovered them performing self-examinations. I was there to tell them that the routine mammogram had shown a suspicious area of calcification and that I would need to refer them to a specialist. I was there when the happy results came back showing that a lump was a cyst or that it was benign. I was there when the results showed cancer and they would have to undergo surgery, radiation or chemotherapy, or all three. I saw women who had undergone breast-cancer surgery years earlier and were now grandmothers. But somehow, I never thought that breast cancer would happen to me.

Several experiences with breast cancer from my medical practice stuck with me over the years. The first occurred when I was a medical student studying surgery in the 1970s. These were the days when a woman would be anesthetized for biopsy of a breast lump and might wake up either with a lumpectomy or a mastectomy, depending on whether the surgeon found cancer or not. The woman went to sleep not knowing whether her breast would be there or not when she awoke.

I vividly remember a preoperative ward round with a consultant surgeon, one of the top surgeons in his field in Western Australia. He was personable enough and well-meaning, and he was technically very competent; but like many of his era, he had a somewhat distant bedside manner. He would walk into the patient's room with a retinue of residents, registrars, nurses, and medical students. He would talk briefly with the patient and then be on to the next "case."

On that particular day, we all trouped into the room of a woman who was scheduled for biopsy and possible mastectomy the next day. During the preoperative visit, the surgeon sat on her bed, pointed to her left breast, and said to her, "You have a little bit of 'mischief' there and we will take care of that for you tomorrow." That was all he said. The registrar and resident had admitted her to the ward and had no doubt spoken to her about the operation, but that was the extent of the surgeon's conversation that day.

I was a young medical student at the time, and I remember being absolutely appalled that he had referred to her probable breast cancer as a "bit of mischief." Tomorrow she would wake up after the surgery either with or without a breast. A fellow female medical student and I discussed it at length. The surgeon had meant well—it was simply his style of speech and the kind of medicine that was practiced in those days. It would have taken a lot of courage for this woman to speak up in front of a hospital room full of students and residents, perhaps to ask a question or ask about her options. At least he had not embarrassed her by examining her in front of everyone, as often happened.

I spoke to this woman later that day. She was a young mother and housewife and clearly very worried. But if the surgeon had not talked to her about what was happening, how could I, a young medical student, speak to her about the unspoken?

The next day, I was present in the operating room when the breast biopsy showed carcinoma. I was scrubbed and present with the surgeon, and another doctor, as she underwent a modified radical mastectomy. I was not there when she woke up to be told that she had lost her breast.

The second incident occurred several years later. I recall a conversation with a plastic surgeon I worked for during my internship in that field. I greatly respected him and had seen his excellent work in breast reconstruction. He would also take the time to talk with his patients and get to know them. One day I was standing opposite him, assisting as he operated on a patient with breast cancer.

Our conversation turned to the statistics on outcomes of different treatment options for breast cancer, and I asked him, "If I come to you with a breast lump and the biopsy shows that it is cancer, would you do a lumpectomy instead of a mastectomy?" He said that of course he would—the research was beginning to show that the statistical outcome with lumpectomy and radiation was just as good as with mastectomy.

Somehow, a light went on in my head and I felt relief wash over me. I came away from the conversation with a very clear concept in my mind: if I ever developed a breast lump that turned out to be cancerous, I would have a lumpectomy and radiation unless there were compelling reasons to do otherwise. For some reason, it was reassuring to me to hear him say this at a time when many other surgeons were still pressing their patients to have radical mastectomies.

Finally, I thought of Cheryl. She first came to see me one afternoon after seeing the head of surgery at one of the major teaching hospitals in our state. Within the last year she had had a mastectomy, and recently she had begun complaining of stomach tenderness and indigestion. The surgeon had examined her and done some blood tests but could find nothing. He said that he could not really help her and made an appointment to see her again in three months. She was not satisfied.

On her way home from that appointment, she stopped into my surgery, which was in a small shopping center about five minutes from where she lived. By chance, she saw my name, Neroli, on the door and thought that it was unusual. After finding out that I was a woman, she asked for an appointment and waited until I could see her a little later in the day. I talked with her for quite a while. She shared that she was worried that the cancer may have spread. I examined her and felt that she could indeed have secondary tumors in the abdomen, so I ordered a CT scan. When the result came back later that day, I had to tell her that the cancer had spread to the liver. I sent her back to the surgeon.

That was the beginning of a relationship that only ended with Cheryl's death. I promised that I would help her through her illness, come what may. Over a period of about a year, although she was mostly treated at the hospital, I saw her in my practice and visited her at home between her hospital and outpatient visits. I saw her through the effects of chemotherapy and took care of her during the final months before she passed on. I cared for her at home with the help of a hospice nurse so that she did not have to be hospitalized.

I got to know Cheryl very well. I learned all about her life, her family, what her illness meant to her, and what a difficult path she had to walk. Sometimes at the end of a visit she would offer me a coffee and we would talk about the deeper things of life. What was it like to die? Would there be pain, and what could we do about it? Did I believe in an afterlife? She would call on a regular basis about a physical symptom or for a prescription, but we both knew that often it was a means to be able to talk and ask questions. In many ways, she was lonely and did not have people who really understood what was happening to her. She was worried about her two teenage sons and what would happen to them. She wondered how much time she had left.

As her health started to decline, I did something that I would not normally do with a patient. My sister and I took Cheryl shopping. I have always found shopping to be a great means of escape. I can completely lose myself in a department store or mall, and time just flies. Even if I don't buy anything, I just love to window shop and try things on. Cheryl really wanted to do some normal things and take a break from her routine. So, on the spur of the moment, I invited her to come shopping in a few days, and she was delighted to accept. She had lost her hair due to chemotherapy and she tired very easily. She suffered from the ulcers in her mouth and other physical symptoms that cancer patients know all about, but she was very excited to go shopping with us.

When we went to pick her up, she was all made up and dressed, ready to go, in the smart wig that she usually didn't wear because it was scratchy and she didn't like it. She was wearing an attractive leisure suit, something that many cancer patients adopt because they are so comfortable. We had a happy evening at a local market and mall, buying various things that we did not really need. She bought a jogging suit on sale and encouraged me to buy one too. (After she passed on, I could never wear it without thinking of her with sadness.) By the time we sat down to eat, she was getting tired, and we took her straight home after the meal. The next few days she was exhausted, but she was very happy that she had gone with us. It was the first and last time we went shopping together. I felt a little guilty that she was so tired, yet I think the shopping expedition did her more good than all the other "therapy" she had been getting.

I was with Cheryl just hours before her passing. I had returned from an overseas trip and we had said goodbye before I left, just in case she passed on before I returned. Her mother called when I was still sleeping, trying to get over the jet lag. She said that I must come soon, because Cheryl would not last long. I was surprised that she was still with us and hurried over to see her. She had declined rapidly and was now just skin over bone. She was unconscious most of the time, but when I told her that I was there, she smiled and tried to sit up. She rose up off the pillow for a few seconds and held my hand. I gave her a small gift of a heart-shaped rose-quartz pendant that I had bought for her on my trip. She was so happy to see me, and then she fell back onto the bed and lapsed back into unconsciousness.

I had told her that if the angels came for her, she should go with them. Her entire family was gathered around her. But she had waited for me to return, and for some reason I felt bad about that. I stayed a little while and then returned home to sleep. She passed that night, and I returned to sign the death certificate and comfort the family. She left a husband and two teenage boys, a sister and mother, all of whom loved her deeply. I attended her funeral. She was wearing the rose-quartz heart around her neck.

To go through an illness with someone in such an intimate and personal way is very moving. In a very real sense, I lived through that illness with Cheryl. It was a draining experience, one that affected me for a long time. For years after her death, she would often come into my mind.

After seeing her undergo chemotherapy, I remember thinking that I would never do it myself. It seemed that she was dealing with its devastating side effects even when there was really no hope of recovery. And she took it because she so wanted to live.

Ten years later, I was the one with breast cancer. I remembered all of those experiences with Cheryl. I could very easily imagine myself walking the same path—dying at a young age, leaving behind my husband and those I loved. And I wondered if I would have the courage to go through all she had experienced.

As time passed, I found, as do many other cancer patients, that you do what you need to do. God seems to give you a courage that you did not know you possessed. I was grateful for the lessons that Cheryl's life had taught me.

LEARN FROM THE JOURNEY OF OTHERS BUT REMEMBER

THAT THE JOURNEY THROUGH CANCER IS YOUR OWN.

CHAPTER 3

CHOICES TO BE MADE

In my previous consultation with the surgeon, I had told him that I needed some time to think about my choices and that once I was sure and had made up my mind, I could go with that choice. He preferred that I move quickly but told me that I had up to a month to make a decision as to whether or not to have a mastectomy. In other words, I had time to do my homework, find out my options, and make my choices.

I called the surgeon that he recommended for a second opinion, explained my situation, and asked for the first available appointment. The earliest he could fit me in was in two weeks! I found it amazing that I was supposed to consider having a mastectomy on Monday, but a second opinion could wait for two weeks. Nevertheless, I was prepared to take my time to make the right choice, so I settled in to wait for the appointment. In the meantime, my surgeon had arranged for me to see an oncologist whose monthly visit to our town happened to be the next Tuesday.

The oncologist was very helpful. He knew that I had been a doctor but that I was not practicing medicine now, and he spent over an hour with me explaining my options and his recommendations. Peter and I talked with him about chemotherapy and radiation. He answered all my questions, and I was receptive to the answers, more able to take them in now that I was getting used to the idea of having breast cancer. The chemotherapy frightened me the most, but I was amazed to find that after seeing the oncologist I actually felt that that chemotherapy was doable. I left the appointment in an optimistic mood—the upswing of the yo-yo of my emotions.

Here's what I had to say in my journal about that day.

Journal Entry
February 4, 1999

Yesterday was a turning point. I felt much more hopeful and more able to cope with the darkness and depression that had been pressing in on me. At 9:00 A.M. I went to see the oncologist with Peter. I spent one hour with him, and he was kind and helpful. He seemed quite optimistic, and the chemotherapy did not sound as bad as it used to be ten years ago. I took notes and he gave me a lot of good information. He gave me his phone number in case I wished to call or had further questions. It really helps to talk to specialists and get their opinions. He showed me the X-rays and shook my hand and said that I can have a very good outcome.

That same day, I felt I had enough energy to start a three-ring binder for all my results, my conversations with people, and all the research that I have begun to gather. Beginning a notebook helps me to feel some semblance of order in a time of chaos. I put a picture of Mary, the Queen of the Angels, on the front of the binder.

Looking back, that oncologist did me a great favor. He gave me hope, and hope is the beginning of healing. He was the first person in the medical profession to actually express hope, to speak about "a very good outcome." I did not realize until he said those words how desperate I was to hear them. Whether it was based on fact or not, I did not really care—I almost loved him for it.

I do think that he is a careful doctor and that he meant what he said. But there is a difference between the approach of a surgeon (who sees you for a major crisis in your life, or the averting of one, and then moves on) and an oncologist, who has a relationship throughout your illness. This doctor could take the larger view, beyond immediate decisions about treatment.

I repeated his words several times so that they would sink in. I understood in a very personal way the impact a doctor can have on a patient and on how one feels about one's illness.

As well as giving me hope, this oncologist had begun to alleviate one of my greatest fears by explaining the advances in treating the side effects of chemotherapy. I wasn't sold, but a door was open that had been closed before.

Nevertheless, for most of the period following my initial diagnosis, I felt overwhelmed. My life had completely changed in almost every way. I found it hard to concentrate. I did not feel like eating. Sometimes I slept for hours; at other times I could not sleep at all. I spent a lot of time in prayer and meditation, asking for guidance as to what to do. I felt that I had a hollow, painful space where my heart was. I was often frightened, but then felt peace again when I prayed and did my spiritual work. I cried a lot and did not feel like talking to people except those who knew me very well—and those were just a handful. Peter was my mainstay. I hugged him a lot.

People in my community heard of my diagnosis and started sending me all kinds of helpful information—books, videos, products, and reading material. Peter was the one who searched the Internet, made phone calls, and researched treatment options for me. I felt unable to do it, as though it was suddenly beyond me. I was a capable person, and had performed a job that entailed a great deal of responsibility, but now making a phone call seemed to be more than I could handle. All I could do was read the material Peter found for me.

My journal recorded my thoughts and feelings as well as my options and progress. My three-ring binder of information soon grew to three binders. I read through the growing pile of material about breast cancer that Peter had printed out for me. I started a separate binder for all of the personal medical information that was beginning to accumulate as well as medical bills and insurance records.

Peter screened my calls and visitors and made all my appointments. I do not know what I would have done without him. He seemed to know exactly what to do. He gave hugs and kisses, held me when I needed to be held, sat with me when I cried, listened when I wanted to talk, encouraged me when I needed it, made me laugh even when I felt that I could never, ever be happy again, and he was always there to help me take the next step. He discussed all the treatment options with me in detail, but he let me know that the final decision was mine and he would support me in whatever choices I made.

Gradually, certain things began to solidify, and I began to be very sure of one thing: I wanted to combine the best of traditional and alternative treatments to create a treatment plan that was right for me.

Four or five months before my diagnosis, I had seen an advertisement in a women's health magazine for Cancer Treatment Centers of America (CTCA). Something happened when I read that ad, which showed a young woman named Julie playing a violin. The caption said, "A thousand concerts ago, I had breast cancer." The words touched me. She'd "had" breast cancer. That meant that she did not have it any more. She was young, like me, and she was fighting and winning. A little voice inside my head said, "If I ever get anything like that, I will go there."

Now, several months later, I could barely recall anything through the fog that my once-agile brain had become. I did not even remember seeing the ad until Peter found the website of CTCA. Then I remembered the logo in the advertisement, and Julie, the violinist. That same day, a girlfriend called and left a message on my answering machine. It was the toll-free number for CTCA. I felt an unseen hand guiding me.

Peter called CTCA and talked to one of their customer representatives. A package of information arrived the next day. I liked what

I read. They had the best of medical, surgical, and oncology care, with state-of-the-art equipment. I saw pictures of the medical staff and read about their background and training as well as the treatment facility. They administered chemotherapy in fractionated doses over several days to minimize side effects. They had a mind-body program. They used nutrition to help their patients fight cancer. They had pastoral care and counseling programs. They had naturopathic physicians on staff. It was just what I was looking for.

Peter called again. They would fly us out to their center in Zion, Illinois, for an evaluation. They would pay for the flights and pick us up at the airport. When could we come? Tomorrow?

We gathered my medical records, X-rays, mammograms, and biopsy samples and flew to Zion. The next day, we checked in at the oncology intake office of the CTCA hospital, Midwestern Regional Medical Center.

I saw one of the surgical oncologists. I immediately liked him. Coincidentally, he had relatives in Perth, and we talked about that. He was capable and caring. I said that I wanted not to have a mastectomy, if at all possible. He said that it was "very reasonable to conserve the breast"—a careful choice of words. He had my mammograms and biopsy reviewed by their specialists and then recommended a lymph-node biopsy. We asked a lot of questions and talked to him for some time. He said he would probably recommend chemotherapy and radiation once the results were available. I liked him and trusted him and I felt it best to have the lymph-node surgery there, at a larger center that specialized in this kind of surgery and did a lot of it, rather than back home. So we scheduled a lymph-node biopsy the next day.

Before seeing the surgeon I spoke with Elizabeth Crane, the director of the mind-body program at the hospital. The program is based on the emerging science of psychoneuroimmunology (PNI) and is designed to enhance your fight against cancer by mobilizing your immune system to assist you. Elizabeth was to become my counselor during my association with CTCA. A lot of things were coming up for me very fast, and as soon as I settled into the comfortable chair in her office I burst into tears. I began to realize some of the pressure I was under.

Elizabeth also gave me an audio tape to use prior to surgery or during chemotherapy or radiation and a tape for general relaxation. She explained that tension and stress depress the immune system and that relaxation and breathing can assist the immune system to fight the cancer. She came to see me before and after my surgery to help me go over mind-body relaxation techniques.

After seeing the surgeon I saw the nutritionist, who went over the details of the clinic's nutritional advice for cancer patients. I was surprised to find that the menus at the hospital included organically grown food. I soon found out that their meals were healthier and even tasted better than those in the hospitals where I had worked. After this there was a battery of tests. I had a CT scan and a bone scan, both of which were negative. The lymph-node surgery was uneventful. The next day the surgeon told me that my lymph nodes were clear.

I was delighted to hear that there was no evidence of the cancer having spread. But in some ways, what really lifted my spirits was when my surgeon said that he thought that I did not need to have a mastectomy. The oncological radiologists were not too concerned about the other areas of calcification in the breast. They thought that these might disappear with radiation and that they could reassess them once that was completed. And after examining the tissue samples from my local hospital, the team of specialists found that the tumor, which had appeared to be two centimeters in diameter on the ultrasound, was only one centimeter in diameter. They felt that the margins of the lumpectomy were adequate and that I did not need any further excision of breast tissue. They would have been happier with somewhat wider margins around the tumor, but they thought what had been done would be adequate if followed up with radiation therapy. If there were a recurrence in that breast, then I would have to have a mastectomy.

At this point they considered my cancer stage I—a lump smaller than two centimeters, no cancer cells in the lymph nodes, and no signs of the cancer having spread to the bone or other organs. Some good news at last, and statistically, as Peter liked to remind me, a 90 percent chance of being cancer-free in five years.

I was very happy, but still cautious—I still had a long way to go. I went to see the radiation oncologist, who recommended radiation therapy. I was discharged after twenty-four hours, and I was scheduled to visit with the oncologist when I returned in three weeks, after the surgical wound had healed. If I decided to take the chemotherapy, I could begin the course of treatment then. I had many things to think about and more choices to make—but one step at a time.

The next day I flew home from Zion with a small drain under my arm, which allowed the excess lymph fluid to drain from the surgical site. I was given exercises to do for my arm to prevent stiffness once the area had healed.

The surgeon had assured me that I was very unlikely to get lymphedema, since he had only sampled a few lymph nodes. I did have numbness in my armpit and on the inside of my upper arm. He told me that the surgery I had undergone often does involve cutting some of the nerves under the arm and I had a fifty-fifty chance of sensation returning within six months. In my case, this did not happen, and I still have a numb area. This was annoying at first, but now does not bother me at all.

The surgeon had told me that I could remove the drain myself after it stopped collecting fluid for twenty-four to forty-eight hours. He knew that I had been a doctor and trusted me to do it, and so I said I would. I did not want to disappoint him, and I was back in doctor mode—sure, no problem. In retrospect, it would have been better to stay in patient mode and go to a doctor to have the drain removed, but I was not really up to facing my local surgeon yet. I thought he might not be too happy with my going to another facility and having surgery there.

When I returned home, I removed the drain a couple of days after it stopped collecting fluid. But then, as sometimes happens, I had some swelling a few days later. The lymph fluid began to accumulate under the skin at the surgical site. It was swollen and uncomfortable, which made sleeping awkward, and I was worried that there might be an infection or some other problem. I was back in patient mode and second-guessing everything. Had I done the right thing? Was everything okay? I called my sister, the surgeon, in Australia, and then I called the hospital. My case manager was not particularly worried and told me I could have the fluid drained by my local surgeon.

I returned to the local clinic to see the surgeon who had performed my lumpectomy. I liked and respected him and hoped that he would support my choices or at least understand them. He examined me and agreed that the fluid under the arm needed to be drained. This did not hurt at all, because he inserted the needle into the area that was numb.

I told him that I had decided against the mastectomy, that I had had a lymph-node biopsy and was most likely going to return to Illinois for chemotherapy and radiation because I liked their holistic approach and the complementary treatments they offered. The surgeon did not hide his opinion that I had made the wrong decision in not having a mastectomy. I was sad about this. I rather naively brought him literature from CTCA that explained their approach, but he was not really interested in reading it. I felt really awful, as if I had let him down. But I knew that it was the right decision for me, and I was going to stick with it unless new information led me to a different path.

That same day, I also saw an internist at the same clinic. Even if I decided to go ahead with the radiotherapy and chemotherapy at Zion, I might still need to see someone locally from time to time, and CTCA had suggested that I find a local physician to take me on as a patient. Meeting this doctor was not a pleasant experience. He thought it was a waste of money to travel such long distances when I could have "the same treatment here." I tried to explain their holistic approach, but he was not interested or simply did not understand. He even handed back to me the literature from CTCA that I brought for him. He said that he would take me on, because if I had chemotherapy, I might need blood transfusions or treatment for infections or other complications.

He also told me that he had worked at a large and extremely well-known cancer institute on the East Coast. He painted a pretty grim picture and even said that he had seen people go to the larger centers and end up dying without their family beside them. This was a very depressing scenario. At this point I was feeling bad and thought the doctor was being insensitive. My husband was going with me for my hospital visits and treatments, so I was not going to "die alone." In fact, I said to myself, "I am not going to die! What does he know?"

Years later, this doctor had his own tests to pass. He developed throat cancer and underwent surgery, chemotherapy and radiation at a larger center. He also became a changed man—now much more understanding and compassionate towards his patients.

As it turned out, I had my weekly blood tests done at the local hospital. They sent the results to my oncologist at CTCA and this local doctor, but I never did need to see him. I did not have any complications from the chemotherapy.

I called Peter after these appointments, shocked and surprised at the attitude that I had encountered. This doctor was the first one who had talked about me dying. It seemed that he did not understand that I wanted to live—not lay down and die before my time. But in spite of everything, I think he did me a favor. I decided that this *wasn't* going to happen if there was anything I could do about it. For the first time, I really felt like fighting.

I started digging into those piles of research and going to bookstores to look for any book that I could find on breast cancer or cancer in general—traditional or complementary. And I settled down to read and read and read. I also took the time to cook healthy meals for myself, get lots of rest, and do the relaxation exercises. (I was very nervous at the thought of chemotherapy and radiation.) I also spent a set amount of time each day doing my spiritual work. I started to feel that things were looking up and began to feel a little better—and more in the driver's seat.

Back in Zion, three weeks later, my oncologist recommended four to six rounds of chemotherapy treatments at four-week intervals, followed by radiation therapy. He also recommended a five-year course of Tamoxifen. He explained that the statistics show that chemotherapy is helpful for later-stage patients, but since the survival rates are very high with stage-I breast cancer, a very large sample size would be needed to determine whether chemotherapy was beneficial for these patients, and these studies had not yet been completed.

Extrapolating from studies on later-stage cancer, he could say that chemotherapy would probably be helpful for me, but he couldn't point to any studies to prove this, so the decision would have to be mine. He told me to take my time and think about it. If I had more questions or wanted to talk some more, I could page him. I was grateful that he took the time to explain everything, and also that he wasn't putting pressure on me. He was allowing me to make a freewill choice.

In spite of myself, I felt moved to have the chemotherapy. Even though it was a very frightening prospect, I felt that it was the right thing to do. I considered many factors. One was that I was premenopausal, and the disease can be more aggressive in premenopausal women. However, the one factor that tipped the balance in my decision was actually a spiritual and not a medical one.

Our Higher Self often finds ways of communicating with us when we need answers, and my Higher Self got through to me in a very vivid dream shortly after my lymph-node surgery. Normally I do not make an important decision on the strength of a dream, but this one was real, and I understood immediately what it meant.

I dreamed that the results of the lymph-node biopsy had shown that three nodes were invaded with cancer. When I awoke, I just knew that although the tests had shown no evidence of it, the cancer had already spread into the lymph system and possibly into the blood as well. This possibility is the reason that cancer patients are followed up so carefully, especially in the first few years. Those cells that spread are only microscopic and may not show in tests. The patient may receive a clean bill of health after initial treatment, only to find that those cells have started to multiply and appear as secondary tumors months or years later. As a result of the dream, I felt I knew something that the doctors didn't know—that the cancer had already spread. Strangely, there was no fear in this knowledge. It was just a fact that I needed to face.

The decision about chemotherapy was probably one of the most difficult I have had to make in this life. As a doctor, I knew the risks and potential side effects. I had also seen my patients go through it, and I had promised myself I would never do it. Nevertheless, after a lot of prayer, thought, and discussion with Peter, I called the oncologist, and we began that afternoon.

The motto of Cancer Treatment Centers of America is, "Winning the fight against cancer every day." At first, the concept of "fighting" the cancer was not one I could really identify with. I did not think of myself as a cancer-fighter. If I "lost the fight against cancer," would I be a loser? I did not think so. But now that I have been through the cancer journey, I understand what they mean. However, I also understand that not everyone wants to fight cancer, and not everyone should.

I saw this in my medical practice and my work as a minister. There are those who know that their time has come to leave this world and that a better world awaits them. They know that chemotherapy is not for them— it would just make their last days more difficult. Others are delighted that chemotherapy gives them a chance to extend their lives and have renewed opportunity to finish certain cycles and projects, to mend relationships, or simply to have more time with family and friends.

In the end, chemotherapy is a very personal decision.

HANG ON TO HOPE. HOPE IS THE BEGINNING OF HEALING. EVEN A GRAIN OF HOPE CAN GROW AND FLOURISH.

CHAPTER 4

CHEMOTHERAPY AND RADIATION

Chemotherapy was the most difficult part of the entire cancer experience for me, as it is for most cancer patients. But it was certainly doable. It had improved tremendously from what I had known ten years earlier in my medical practice. Nevertheless, I look forward to a time when no one will have to go through it.

CTCA administers fractionated-dose chemotherapy. Instead of receiving one injection over about twenty minutes or so, the patient receives a diluted dose, distributed over five days. The purpose of this is to minimize the side effects of the drugs without reducing their effectiveness against cancer cells.

I chose to have the chemotherapy administered via a central line that was inserted into the large vein under my collarbone each time I visited the hospital. The procedure was performed by my surgeon under local anesthetic. I used to be pretty good at putting them in when I was a doctor, but being on the other end of the needle was a different experience. The central line saves wear and tear on the patient's veins—

especially helpful for someone with hard-to-find veins like mine.

Like most patients, I do not like foreign things going into my body, and I always breathed a sigh of relief when the line was removed after five days. Nevertheless, repeated needles for injections and blood samples are not pleasant, and I was grateful to have this alternative.

The first time I had chemotherapy, they kept me in the hospital so they could watch for adverse reactions. For me, this first treatment was the hardest one of all.

I was hooked up to an infusion pump that delivered small doses of the three chemotherapy drugs. The pump could be plugged into a wall outlet or it could run on its battery for about an hour, enabling me to walk around the hospital if I wanted to, pulling the IV pole with me. Different combinations of chemotherapy drugs are given at different rates; mine was set to be delivered over a period of eight to ten hours each day for five days per session. At the end of the day, the pump was disconnected and the line was flushed with a heparin solution to prevent blood clots from blocking the line.*

After the first round of treatment as an inpatient, staying in the hospital overnight, I was able to receive subsequent rounds as an outpatient. During the day, I would sit with other patients in one of the chemotherapy rooms. We had comfortable reclining chairs, and we could talk and have visitors. After the daily treatment, I would go to my hotel room.

Peter was able to juggle his work schedules so that he could come with me to all of the sessions. It was a tremendous support to have him there, and I would not have wished to go through the experience of chemotherapy alone. However, I also met people who did very well by themselves.

During the course of treatment, blood tests were taken every day. Once the treatment was completed and I flew home, I had weekly blood

---

* Since I received my treatment in 1999, there have been some significant advances in chemotherapy delivery. Many hospitals now offer continuous infusion, in which chemotherapy agents are delivered continuously over a period of one or more days. This is delivered by a small portable pump that the patient wears at home.

tests at my local hospital. (Chemotherapy affects the immune system, and it is important to check that immune function is not depressed too much.) The results were faxed to CTCA.

The most common side effects of chemotherapy are nausea and vomiting. For me these passed fairly quickly, thanks to the vast improvements in antinausea medication now available. Although I rarely vomited during treatments, I never was hungry and disliked eating while the chemotherapy drugs were going into my body. I experienced a fairly constant state of sublevel nausea—not too bad, but not pleasant—but this was nothing like the nightmares that I had seen with cancer patients. I did not lose weight, and my appetite was only affected during the five days of chemotherapy each month.

After the first round, I was very tired for about a week. After the others, I was tired for two or three days, and then my energy level returned to normal, or even better than normal. I had one episode of bad constipation. I lost about two thirds of my hair. I also went through menopause early as a result of the chemotherapy.

All in all, I felt that it was not a bad result, in some ways better than I expected. In between chemotherapy sessions I felt and looked well—probably better than I had in years. I worked hard to keep my body in good condition to receive the chemotherapy, and I have documented the details in chapter 15, "Getting through Chemo." I think it was this hard work, as well as the fractionated-dose delivery, that enabled me to do so well.

Before the fourth round of chemotherapy, I had decided that this was to be the last for me. My body and my heart told me that I did not need more than four. (I will explain more about this decision later.) I consulted with my oncologist prior to the fourth treatment, and he wanted me to have two more rounds. He said, "Why not do the final two, as you are doing so well?" I explained that I felt that this was enough and that it was precisely because I was doing so well that I did not want any more. When I told him how I felt, he said that he respected my decision and could support it.

After the chemotherapy, there was a break of several weeks, and then it was time for radiation. I decided to have the radiotherapy at CTCA. The radiation oncology wing had opened less than a year earlier, and they had the latest and most advanced computer-controlled equipment, which could deliver concentrated doses of radiation to the target area with minimum exposure to surrounding areas. I could have received radiation at a local hospital in Montana, but they did not have the same advanced equipment, and it would have meant a two-hour journey each day from home to the hospital and back.

The specialist recommended thirty-three days of treatment, five days a week for six and a half weeks. I rented a room in a house across the street from the hospital. I felt very well while I was there and enjoyed my stay. There was some redness in the area being irradiated for about three weeks. Around week four I got a little tired, but I do not feel that was related to the radiation as much as a weekend business trip back home, where I did not get much sleep.

The treatment was only for a short period each day, so I was able to meet with staff and other patients and attend the programs the hospital conducted. For many reasons, I felt it was worth the investment of time and energy it took for me to be there rather than have the treatment in my local center.

I completed my treatment and felt very well—in fact, much better than before the cancer was diagnosed. I returned to work, and my career took a different direction. I continue to have regular checkups.

In summary: I had a one-centimeter cancerous tumor in my right breast, adenocarcinoma, stage I. There was no evidence of spread to the lymph nodes or elsewhere in the body.

I underwent two surgeries—lumpectomy and lymph-node biopsy. I went through four cycles of chemotherapy and thirty-three days of radiotherapy at a center that combined these treatments with complementary therapies. I made use of nutrition as well as naturopathy. I used a variety of herbs and supplements and a number of other natural healing methods. I embarked upon an exercise program. I relied heavily upon prayer and spiritual support as well as mind-body techniques and visualization. I also worked with a clinical psychologist.

Eight years later I had a local recurrence in the muscle near the shoulder, most likely due to a dose of topical, localized estrogen which was inadvertently given to me by a well-meaning gynecologist. My oncologist said that my breast cancer was very estrogen sensitive, and even the small amount of estrogen that was absorbed systemically could have triggered the recurrence.

I had an opportunity to reread and reapply the principles in this book. After another round of surgery and radiation, I am on a daily dose of an anti-estrogen medication. I am once again cancer-free and even more diligent about taking care of myself.

People often ask what helped the most. I am hesitant to answer that question, because I feel that no one thing was the sole reason for my success. I took an active role in putting together the program for the treatment of my illness, and I think it was all of these things working together. My life has definitely changed for the better through the whole experience.

CHAPTER 5

WHAT I LEARNED ABOUT MYSELF

One morning, I looked outside and it was raining. It dawned on me then that I did not need to wait any longer for a rainy day to be able to do those things that I wanted and needed to do for myself. My rainy day was here.

Dr. Patrick Quillin, director of nutrition at CTCA, says, "Of all risk factors for breast cancer in the hundreds of patients I have worked with, stress is the most common. Almost all experienced a traumatic event such as divorce or a loved one's death about a year or two prior to their diagnosis. So relax and be yourself. Don't put excess emphasis on the past or the future. Practice nontoxic stress relief, such as prayer, meditation, exercise, music, talking to friends, and writing in your journal. Take time each day to care for yourself."[1]

I learned many things about myself in the course of cancer treatment. Some of these things were surprising. Some were not new, but I was somehow not willing or able to put them into practice in a meaningful way until I got cancer. Cancer was the catalyst for change.

Some of these learnings were very personal. Others I am able to share.

Here are a few flowers grown in the garden of self, after my rainy days.

- I am learning to deal with my tendency to take care of others at the expense of myself. I am learning not to be everyone else's caregiver. I am commending others to God's care and the care of the angels, even as I give myself to the care of the angels.
- I am learning the difference between sympathy and compassion. Sympathy pulls me down but true compassion uplifts me and those I am seeking to help.
- I am learning a true sense of responsibility towards myself and others.
- I am learning to take care of and nurture myself. I am trying to do something comforting or which pleases me each day. It can be a small act of kindness to myself. It can be as simple as a warm scented bath with candles at the end of the day. It can be a walk at dusk when I consciously let go of any problems. It may be a treat, such as buying a small bouquet of fresh flowers or some other thing that delights my senses.
- I am listening to my body to find out what it wants me to do to stay healthy, and I am listening to my heart so that I know what course my life should take.
- I am learning to take delight in small things. Before, I barely noticed the colors of the leaves on the trees. Now, I can lie on the grass and watch the way the sunlight comes through the clouds.
- I am learning better ways to cope with stress. I can now take small amounts of time out of my day to de-stress and take care of myself. I am consciously letting go of tensions and old habits, over-concern and worry.
- I am learning to watch my thoughts. I consciously weed out of my garden of thoughts the ones that are not helpful.
- I am learning to set loving boundaries and to say no to things and people that are not helpful or positive for me.
- I am learning that I do not have to rush and that life is not always a race against time. I can take time to breathe deeply in stressful

situations.

- I am taking time to smell the roses (literally).
- I am liking myself more and more each day. I am learning to visualize myself as whole and healthy.

Here is something I wrote in my journal:

I am starting to develop a profound sense of peace and a greater and greater awareness of the power of the spiritual path. Even though I was aware of many elements of the spiritual path and practiced them before, now it is different and deeper. I can see that for a long time I have not been truly living—I have merely existed.

As I look back, I see that I have had an uneasy feeling for months and felt a pain in my heart many times, and underneath, a sense of depression. Sometimes I would throw up in the mornings for no apparent reason—just sick to my stomach—about what? I would ignore it and keep going.

At the same time I craved balance, wholeness, meditation, exercise, proper diet, and self-nurturing. I had taken to having baths in bubbles with candles for relaxing and meditating. I was taking weekends off, but it was taking me a long time to recover from the week. I kept buying more and more books on healing and psychology and spirituality and wholeness. I wanted to spend more time praying and pursuing the spiritual path

There was a train coming straight for me, but I could not see it. I can now see the handwriting on the wall that I could not see then. I can also see that God was preparing me. I am so grateful.

SIMPLE THINGS TO DO WHEN YOU FEEL STRESSED ABOUT CANCER

✓ Take some deep breaths
✓ Pray and meditate
✓ Go for a walk or do yoga or some form of exercise
✓ Listen to uplifting music
✓ Talk to a friend or a family member
✓ Write in your journal

SECTION II

My Approach to Cancer

CHAPTER 6

A ROAD MAP FOR THE JOURNEY

A s a doctor, I thought that I knew a lot about cancer—until I got it myself. I found out that there is far more to cancer than diagnosis and treatment. It is not just a medical condition: it is something that impacts your whole life.

You are more than your body, and you can't separate your body from the other aspects of yourself (at least, not while you are alive). Your mind, emotions, your soul and your body are connected and interdependent.

If your car has a problem, you find a good mechanic, pay your money and trust that he will fix it. Sometimes we might wish that we could heal the body this way—go to the doctor and get it "repaired." But your body is not just a machine that you use—and you can't so easily trade it in for a new model if it is no longer working well! Something more is needed, for both doctors and patients.

Doctors go to school for many years to learn how to treat cancer medically. But what about all the other aspects?

More importantly, where is the training course for patients?

Most often we have to learn as we go along, sometimes by trial and error, making our own roadmap as we travel through an unknown land.

Here are the some of the insights that helped me the most on my journey through cancer.

TREAT THE WHOLE PERSON

No one *really* knows what causes cancer. Every day, cells in our body divide and new cells are formed to replace ones that are lost or damaged. Every time a cell divides, it is possible for an abnormal cell to be created. In fact, this happens quite frequently. These abnormal cells can become cancer cells that continue to divide and grow unchecked, eventually forming a cancerous mass or lump.

So why doesn't everyone have cancer?

We can thank our immune system for this. One of the functions of this system is to recognize and deal with abnormal cells.

Although I learned these facts in medical school, I never fully understood their importance until I got cancer myself. The immune system is the key in dealing with cancer, and although we tend to talk about the immune system as if it were a single organ or system, it is really a complex interaction of many organs and systems in the body. Thus, no matter what the location of a particular tumor, cancer is a whole-body disease, and the treatment will be most effective if it addresses the whole body.

Furthermore, as researchers learn more and more about the mind and emotions and their interaction with the body—especially the immune system—they are also discovering how much of a difference treating the whole person makes. (I will be discussing this aspect of healing in chapter 13, "Medicine and the Mind.")

ASSEMBLE YOUR TEAM

When you are looking at the whole person (rather than just a lump of abnormal cells) you realize that healing really is a team effort. The members of the team are fourfold:

1. **You and your body** (including your mind and emotions).

2. **Your doctors, therapists and all those who help with the various aspects of your healing.** You probably won't find a single individual who is an expert in *all* the areas you want to work on, from the spiritual to the emotional to the physical. Instead, you will probably find that there are many different people who can help you in their own areas of expertise. These people will all be a part of your team.

3. **Your family and friends.** People close to you can also be an important part of your team, and they can provide help and support emotionally, spiritually and even physically that doctors, hospitals and professionals are not able to provide.

4. **The force of healing.** Last, but by no means least, is the wonderful force that most of us take for granted. Whatever you call it, this spiritual force is the true source of healing for which everyone else, including yourself, is but an instrument. The force of healing has many names and manifestations, depending on your belief system and your background: the life-force, the light, God in all of his names and manifestations, the angels, and your own spiritual forces, including your guardian angel and Higher Self.

This force is the true head of your team in the spirit realm. However, on this physical plane we call earth, you are the head of the team.

You Are the Head of Your Team

Remind yourself that you are the head of the team when it comes to your health and healing. Many people do not realize this, nor do they think of themselves this way, but you are the one who must make the final decisions.

You can gather around you all kinds of experts and helpers, but in the end, the buck stops with you. You make the choices, and it is your plan that is carried out. (Or if you don't, you allow others to formulate a plan for you—but this is also a choice.)

This concept gives you a lot of freedom, but it also carries a responsibility. I felt additional responsibility as a doctor and a minister, in that people would observe the choices that I made and whatever I did might influence their choices.

Dr. Bernie Siegel was the first person to open my eyes to the concept of taking a very active role in my treatment. I had read his book *Love, Medicine, and Miracles* several years before getting cancer and loved his approach to both cancer and healing. When I got sick I picked it up again, not as a doctor but as a patient.

Dr. Siegel is a pediatric surgeon who practiced in New Haven, Connecticut. Rather than looking at cancer as an illness to be treated, he looked at the *people* who were dealing with cancer—especially those who survived, and most especially those who survived when their cases seemed hopeless. How did these exceptional patients do it? What was different about them?

He found that the people who survived despite the odds against them were often those who actively engaged in determining the course of their treatment. They asked a lot of questions, wanted to know why, had to check things out for themselves before agreeing to anything. Sometimes medical staff saw them as "difficult." But they survived.[1]

I am not suggesting you become a "difficult" patient, but do your own research, ask questions, explore your options. Get in the driver's seat and you are likely to have a better outcome.

You Have Time to Make Your Choices

Before you make a decision about surgery or any other treatment, take the time that you need to research your type of cancer and your treatment options. Often, the decisions you make will have long-lasting effects—and you will be making them at a time of great stress. The stress itself of finding out that you have (or may have) a life-threatening illness makes it very difficult to weigh all the evidence and make decisions, even if this is something you usually do well.

Generally, I have not had a hard time making decisions in my own life, either personally or professionally. I am blessed with what friends, elderly ladies, and fellow doctors would call "common sense." I like to know all the options before making a decision, and I am willing to do the research required to find out what they are. I also do my spiritual homework and then go with what I feel is the right decision.

The decisions I made about my cancer treatment were some of the most difficult I have had to make in this life. I felt the pressure to deal with my breast lump as soon as possible. My medical training taught me to deal with issues as soon as possible and to make decisions quickly and decisively—you need to be able to do this in an emergency room and in anesthesia. However, cancer is a little different. Things develop over weeks and months, rather than minutes, so there is a different timeframe for decisions. There is time to confirm the diagnosis, seek expert opinion (a second one if necessary), and develop a plan.

Some people feel a sense of urgency to "get on with it and to get it behind me." They want their old life back. I certainly had this feeling. It is legitimate to want to know the diagnosis and know exactly what you are dealing with as soon as possible. However, once you know the diagnosis, there is a healthy sense of urgency and a not-so-healthy one, and it is important to distinguish between the two.

The healthy sense of urgency is the instinct of self-preservation, which wants to face the issue head on, and which doesn't want you to fall into denial or procrastination that would allow the disease to progress further.

The unhealthy sense of urgency is the slightly panicked feeling that would cause you to jump at the first "solution" that is offered. It is sometimes communicated by well-meaning family and friends or even well-intentioned medical and surgical teams, who want to "do something" to solve the problem. In my case, the unhealthy sense of urgency was largely self-generated and came from my days in medical practice, when it was the prevailing opinion that the biopsy and surgery be done as soon as possible.

While you don't want to delay unnecessarily, it is not a good idea to let the idea of acting quickly rule your life at this very important time. You do have time to become fully informed and to develop a plan. It was a great relief to me when I realized that I had time to make a thoughtful decision. I believe this allowed me to make better choices and have a better outcome.

You can ask your doctor (as I did) what would be a reasonable length of time in which to research your options and make a decision.

TALK TO THOSE INVOLVED IN YOUR CARE

When you visit the doctor or talk to anyone concerned with your treatment, be sure to take a pen and notepad. Ask questions and take notes, or even tape record the conversation (with their permission).

It can be very helpful to make a list of your questions ahead of time, even the really basic ones. It is surprising how hard it is to think when you are stressed, taking medication, or worried. It is equally hard even to remember what was said. I knew from my own training and experience as a doctor that most patients can only recall one or two things that are said to them in a consultation. Nevertheless, it was a disconcerting to come out of a consultation and not be able to recall the details. The notepad and pen really helped.

Even when I was feeling fine, I still put all my questions in writing so that I could be sure that I did not forget anything. No question is too inconsequential or stupid. It is important to understand all your options and the consequences of the different choices. It tells you a lot about your doctor, too, whether or not he or she is willing to take the time to answer your questions and listen to your concerns and preferences.

I also highly recommend having someone with you. Peter accompanied me to most of my consultations. If I forgot to ask a question, he could prompt me. If I was not feeling or functioning well, he could ask the questions for me. After the consultation, we compared notes and wrote down additional points we remembered while the concepts were still fresh in our minds.

Doctor's visits are often stressful when the stakes are high. Even when your doctor is friendly and helpful, you are also aware that he or she is a busy person, and that can create a certain pressure in itself. In a single visit, you often get the good or bad news in the form of test results, followed swiftly by the recommendation for the next phase of treatment. You have to take in this information, process it, and then ask questions, all in a matter of minutes. And you are often expected to make major decisions about your life as a result all of this input.

One thing that can help is to plan ahead. Think about the possible outcomes and your choices ahead of time. If the result of the biopsy indicates cancer, what will I ask? What if the results are negative? Write down both lists of questions and take them with you.

It can also be helpful to decouple the information-gathering from decision-making. Remember that you do not have to make a decision on the spot. The doctors who treated me often gave test results and information I needed, answered my questions, and then invited me to go away and think about my decision—even if I was ready to make one immediately.

Do Your Research

There are many books available on treatment of cancer, and many specifically about breast cancer. They are often written by knowledgeable people who are experts in their field.

After the biopsy, I hurried off to the local bookstore and sat in one of their easy chairs with a stack of books on breast cancer, all of which I would eventually buy. I read almost everything I could find on breast cancer and its treatment, ranging from the traditional to the bizarre. I have also read a number of biographies and personal accounts of those who survived the breast-cancer experience and wished to share what they learned.

Taking the time to read widely was very helpful for me. Finding out as much as I could gave me a sense of empowerment or control over the situation. Even my prayers could be more specific. I worried less when I knew what was going to happen. I knew that I had researched all of the options and could feel confident in my choices.

If this is your approach, use the Internet, libraries, and bookstores as resources. Start talking to people and take any opportunity to talk to other patients and their families who have been through what you are facing. Read what other patients have written about their experiences. Ask friends, relatives, and coworkers to send you information.

There are many sources of free information. The National Cancer Institute (www.cancer.gov) offers helpful basic information about traditional medical care. The web site for Cancer Treatment Centers of America (www.cancercenter.com) also has a lot of useful information.

I am an avid reader and can quickly digest a book or article; I read with an open mind and write in the margins and at the end of chapters. I am, however, a somewhat critical reader, and I like to make my own evaluations. I evaluated what each author said in light of my own experience. Although I did not always agree with all the comments of each author, I learned from all of them and their different perspectives. And if someone said that this was the way it was for them, it did not mean that it had to be that way for me.

It was especially helpful to read several books when an issue was sensitive or controversial. For example, whether or not to take Tamoxifen was a big question. I found it helpful to read the chapters on this subject in several different books so that I could get a broad perspective. In the end, I decided that it was not for me. Similarly, before radiation and chemotherapy, I compared the notes from several different sources on that subject to remind myself of what they were saying or to remember any tips or keys that others had found useful.

I also went back and reviewed the books from time to time, because even though I had read them from cover to cover, I often found that I did not recall all the details. Sometimes I would just thumb through a book and I would rediscover sections that were helpful with whatever I happened to be going through at the time. Above all, I followed my intuition and weighed the information not only in my mind but also in my heart.

Not everyone has the time or even the inclination to do the kind of research that I did. It is a very individual matter. You will have to decide how much information *you* need to have to make your decisions and feel confident about your choices. For some people, too much detailed information can create a sense of being overwhelmed and make it more difficult to make decisions. For others (and I am definitely in this category) too little information is stressful.

Trust your feelings about how much information you need to feel well-informed. And if you are in the first category, consider enlisting a close friend or family member as your research assistant, whose job will be to gather all the information, make sure nothing has been missed, summarize, and give you what you need to make your choices.

One word of caution: there is a bewildering array of alternative and complementary therapies, and it is easy to get confused very quickly. Don't be overwhelmed. Do your research, but don't feel that you have to follow every bit of advice you receive. Be selective and choose what is right for you. I will talk more about navigating through these choices in chapter 11, "Complementary Medicine."

GET A SECOND OPINION

Even if you think you feel confident about the diagnosis, the treatment choices, and what you want to do, I strongly recommend getting a second opinion, preferably from a specialist. Almost every book or resource that I found said the same thing. It is money well spent, and many insurance programs will cover the full cost of a second opinion. Sometimes it can make a big difference. I have spoken to a number of men and women with cancer who wish that they had gotten a second opinion before acting.

Dr. Isadore Rosenfeld, author of *Second Opinion: Your Comprehensive Guide to Treatment Alternatives,* writes of one person's experience that illustrates this point very well:

> The wife of one of my doctor friends developed severe headaches and attacks of double vision. She consulted a senior neurologist, who, after thorough testing, discovered a brain tumor. The patient asked for and was told the diagnosis. She was advised that surgery was not possible, and her only alternative was radiation, which would shrink the tumor somewhat and alleviate the headaches, but would not cure her. This gallant lady settled her affairs and prepared to live out her last few months in the greatest possible comfort. Her husband, the doctor, knew better than to shop around for another opinion. This was, after all, an open-and-shut case confirmed by an eminent brain specialist.
>
> But the patient was persuaded by a non-medical friend to see someone else. Reluctantly she consulted an equally prestigious neurosurgeon, who agreed with the diagnosis, but not with the treatment or outlook. He felt confident that the tumor could be completely removed.
>
> With nothing to lose, my friend underwent surgery, and it was entirely successful. The tumor was a large one, pressing on her brain. After its removal, her symptoms disappeared and she returned to a normal life in a few weeks. That was fifteen years ago.[2]

Getting a second opinion does not mean that you do not trust the people that you have seen first. There is no single right answer for everyone. Even different specialists may have different recommendations, and in the end, you have to choose what is right for you. Remember, there is nothing to lose by getting a second opinion. If the second opinion agrees with your first, you can still choose where you want to go for treatment.

Unfortunately, many patients feel uncomfortable about talking to their doctor or surgeon about a second opinion for fear of offending or being seen as a difficult patient. This was certainly the case for me. Even with my medical background, or perhaps even because of that background, it took courage for me to tell my surgeon that I wanted a second opinion. It took even more courage for me to return and say that I had chosen to go with the second opinion instead of his recommendation. Here are some of my thoughts about this at the time:

Journal Entry

Rereading Bernie Siegel's book Love, Medicine and Miracles *has given me great insight into the ways that many doctors think and how they feel responsible for others. I also realized how I have made that a part of my life. As I look back, I have felt over-responsible for many situations in my life and the lives of others and have been concerned for everyone's welfare but my own. I was ready to have my breast removed, because, in one sense, I did not want to disappoint the surgeon. Time to change.*

Summoning the courage to get a second opinion was an important part of my healing journey. It also gave me the space I needed to think about my situation in a different way. I went with this second opinion because it felt right. If I had still not been sure at that point, I would have sought a third opinion.

SEE THE EXPERTS

I live near a small town, and I am glad that I went to a larger medical facility that deals primarily with cancer. My sister, an obstetrician, was first to tell me about studies showing that survival rates are lower in smaller centers and smaller towns. In a sense it is not surprising, although I had never really thought about it before.

Another finding in these studies is that doctors in smaller centers tend to prescribe more aggressive treatment. Perhaps less experienced doctors want to feel that they have done everything they can, whereas those who have seen many more cases are more confident in knowing what will really be helpful in a particular case. When the potential side effects of treatment are significant, there can be real value in not over-treating.

I found a lot of value in being able to discuss my situation with people from a center that specialized in cancer treatment. The conversation was at a higher level—they had seen more cases, done more procedures, had more up-to-date information, and had more resources available to them. They were very familiar and comfortable with patients who had problems just like mine.

Of course, you may have an excellent center right where you are, even in a small town. You may have medical staff that you know and trust, and that may well be the right place for you. I have friends with breast cancer who received excellent care locally. They were very pleased with their treatment and the results. It would have been difficult for them and their families if they had had to receive treatment out of town for long periods of time. And of course, there may be the additional costs for travel and accommodation if you go to a larger center.*

There are many factors to consider, and it will always be an individual choice—one that will depend on your particular circumstances. Above all, you need to find medical professionals you can talk to and whom you trust. Your body and your life will be in their hands.

Keep a Journal of Your Experiences and Insights

I have always loved to write and enjoy writing down my experiences from time to time, but I had never kept a journal on a regular basis. However, within a few days of being diagnosed with breast cancer, I felt a need to keep a journal. Much has been written about journaling as a tool for healing, and I thoroughly recommend it.

Sometimes I would use a computer. At other times I would just write with a pad and pen. Whatever method I used, I found that there was something healing about writing down my thoughts and feelings. I would often get new insights on my situation while I was in the flow of

---

* Travel and accommodation expenses for medical treatment, while generally not reimbursed by insurance, may be tax deductible.

writing. Thoughts and impressions are sometimes fleeting, and it was good to capture them on paper as they occurred.

Apart from the healing experience in the process of writing, I found it very helpful to look back over what I had written earlier and see what I was thinking and feeling at the time. I could see where I had made progress and also areas that still needed work that I might have forgotten about.

My journal entries included what doctors and therapists said to me as well as comments from friends and family, especially when what they said moved me. Sometimes a comment or phrase would linger in my mind for a long time—like a talisman or a good luck charm.

I also kept all the letters, cards, and e-mails of support from many sources. I would reread them on the dark days when the sun did not seem to be shining or it was hard going, and they offered insight and inspiration. I even put a few on the refrigerator door so that I could see them every day. It is great to know that you are loved and that friends and coworkers are praying for you and cheering you on.

KEEP A NOTEBOOK OF CANCER RESOURCES

Many cancer patients keep a notebook of resources, and I also found this useful. My notebook had sections for resources about cancer, conventional medical information, and alternative therapies.

People sent me all kinds of information, articles, and helpful hints. As each item arrived, I read it and filed it in the appropriate section. That way options did not just float through my brain with nowhere to lodge. I knew what I had considered and what I had discarded as not workable for me. It gave me a sense of empowerment at a time when my moorings seemed to be shifting wildly.

KEEP A NOTEBOOK OF YOUR MEDICAL PROGRESS

I had a separate notebook to keep track of my medical history. In a three-ring binder I filed results of blood tests, mammograms, scans and X-rays, scheduling of medical appointments, and notes on what the doctor or therapist said at each appointment. I asked for copies of my medical records and filed them also. I took this notebook with me each time I saw a new doctor or therapist. They can do a better job for you if they have all the information they need.

I also kept a chronology of the illness on a separate page in this notebook. I recorded dates of key events, including surgery, chemotherapy, and radiation beginning and end dates. This was often useful. It seemed that there were many times when I had to recount my history.

I kept a page on which I listed the medications or supplements I was taking. Each time I entered the hospital, I had to list these, and it saved a lot of time and energy to have all the information in one place, especially when I was tired or stressed or my brain was not functioning as well as usual.

Medical bills and insurance records seem to roll in very quickly, and I kept another file for these. These financial records can be confusing, and it sometimes feels as if you are drowning in paperwork. I also found that the sight of these bills coming in each week was depressing, even though I knew that most were covered by insurance. If they were all three-hole-punched and filed in order, it was easier to keep track of what had been paid and what hadn't and I didn't have to put so much time and attention on them.

BE PRACTICAL AND DEAL WITH THE REALITY OF YOUR SITUATION

At the time that I was going through the rigors of chemotherapy, I learned of two other women in my church community who were dealing with breast cancer. They died within three days of one another while I was receiving chemotherapy. I talked to one of them several times before she passed on, which brought home the reality of this life-threatening illness even more.

Both women had chosen to receive very little in the way of conventional medical treatment and had used mostly alternative therapies. One of them eventually had a mastectomy, but it was very late. The local tumor on the breast had grown very large, to the size of an orange, and the cancer had already spread throughout her body. I discovered that the same surgeon who removed my breast lump had removed her breast just weeks before. I could understand at that point his sense of urgency that I act decisively and have a mastectomy.

I do not know all the history of these cases or why these women made the choices that they did, nor do I judge them. However, I could not help but wonder if their avoidance of conventional medical treatment contributed to their passing. Their deaths had a profound influence on me and on others in our community, and seeing the progression of their cases in the months before and after my diagnosis spurred me on to pursue all options and to take my healing very seriously.

Join a Support Group

Studies show that women with breast cancer who belong to support groups, even for a period of twelve months, survive longer.[3] I longed to be able to talk to people who had been through what I was going through. However, I have heard of really good support groups and ones that were not so helpful. I was equally sure that I could not afford to spend time with people who were depressed or down as a result of cancer.

My surgeon did not know of any support groups near where I lived, nor could I find one in my local area through the phone book or the Internet. Although they now exist in my area, at the time, the nearest one I could find was three hours away, and that was too far. If you live in a large city, you should be able to find a support group nearby. There are thousands of these groups all over the country.

Some patients start their own support groups and really benefit from the experience. My surgeon had offered to put me in contact with other women in the local area who had dealt with breast cancer and I could have started my own group, but I knew that this would not be good for me at that time. Given my nature, if I was organizing the group I might have soon found myself taking care of the other people at the expense of my own health.

I knew three women in my church community who had battled breast cancer, and I decided to talk to them one-on-one. Their experiences were different and very personal. Two had readily shared their experiences with others. One had considered it a very private matter and had hardly spoken to anyone else. We talked about all kinds of things, and I learned from each of them. We cried together and supported one another.

Finally, when I went to CTCA, I had the opportunity to talk to other patients. During chemotherapy I met many women with breast cancer and patients with different types of cancer. A number of breast cancer patients had similar schedules to mine and we would meet each month.

During the six-and-a-half weeks that I received radiation, there were six other women with breast cancer who were also receiving radiation treatment. Several of us stayed together in a house across the street made available by the hospital at very reasonable rates. We attended exercise classes and programs at the hospital, went on excursions together, and talked a lot about our experiences with cancer. We were a live-in support group.

And yes, our activities did include "shopping therapy"—a visit to a mall or a nearby store to buy something that was on sale or that lifted our spirits and forget about cancer for a while. We also laughed a lot—at ourselves, at the illness, and at the experiences we shared. No one on the outside really knows what it is like to go through cancer, and I felt that a unique bond was formed in our time together.

CHECKLIST: STARTING THE JOURNEY

✓ Treat the whole person. Cancer is a whole-body disease—the most effective treatment program addresses the whole body.

✓ Assemble your team. Your team is you and your body, any health professional involved in your care, family and friends, and whatever you call the spiritual force of healing.

✓ You are the head of your team. Those who actively engage in determining the course of their treatment do better. They are the ones who tend to survive despite the odds.

✓ You have time to make your choices. Your decisions will likely have long lasting effects. In most cases you have time to become fully informed and to develop a plan.

✓ Talk to those involved in your care. Ask questions—true professionals don't mind.

✓ Write down your questions beforehand. And don't forget to take pen and paper to take notes. It is surprising how quickly you can forget what was said.

✓ Take someone with you to appointments, if possible. Compare notes afterwards to get a fuller picture.

✓ Do your research. Don't be overwhelmed, but do enough research so that you can feel you are making fully-informed decisions.

✓ Don't feel that you have to follow every bit of advice you receive. Be selective and choose what is right for you.

✓ Get a second opinion. You have nothing to lose by getting a second opinion and there may be a lot to gain. Even after getting a second opinion, you can still choose where you want to go for treatment.

✓ See the experts. It really does make a difference—survival rates are higher in larger centers that specialize in cancer treatment.

✓ Be practical and deal with the reality of your situation. Pursue all reasonable options and do not ignore the obvious.

✓ Join a support group. People who are in a support group do better.

✓ Don't be burdened by the memory of someone else's experience with cancer. You can learn from other's experiences, but you are walking your own path.

✓ Allow others to help you.

✓ Use a system to keep track of all your information. My system had four categories: (a) a journal for my personal experiences and insights, (b) a three-ring binder for research and resources, (c) another binder for medical test results and notes from meetings with doctors, (d) a file for medical bills and insurance records.

Chapter 7

MAKING THE BEST OF SURGERY

The three primary conventional treatments for cancer are surgery, radiation therapy, and chemotherapy. The specific treatments recommended for a particular patient will vary depending on the type of cancer, how advanced it is at the time of discovery, and many other factors.

If surgery is part of the treatment plan, it is often the first thing that is done. However, for some cancers, radiation and/or chemotherapy may be used first in order to shrink the cancer prior to surgery.

For breast cancer, most traditional treatment plans involve surgery. This may be lumpectomy (surgical removal of just the lump) or mastectomy (removal of the whole breast). In either case some of the lymph nodes under the arm may also be removed to see if cancer has spread beyond the breast itself.

Surgery is often followed by chemotherapy and/or radiation. If a mastectomy is performed, radiation is usually not required unless the cancer has spread beyond the breast. I will devote the remainder of this chapter to the subject of surgery and discuss radiation and chemotherapy in future chapters.

There is an old joke that "minor" surgery is surgery that happens to someone else. A lumpectomy or a lymph-node dissection may be considered minor surgery, but when it's you that is being cut open, it definitely does not feel minor. The good news is that if you do have to undergo surgery, there are things you can do to help get the best outcome.

A good place to start is to know what to expect if you will be having surgery. If you know what will happen, you can do the best job of preparing and working with your body for a good outcome, a swift recovery, and fewer side effects. Most hospitals have information available for patients. There is also a lot of information available for free on the Internet.

With my medical background, I knew what went on in the operating room. Modern surgery and anesthesia are refined and professional, so I was not too concerned about that aspect of my treatment. However, even though I had been there for other women's breast surgeries, you can never really know what it is like to be operated on until it happens to you.

A very useful resource was Peggy Huddleston's book *Prepare for Surgery, Heal Faster: A Guide of Mind-Body Techniques*. Huddleston quotes studies showing that people who prepare for surgery have "less pain, fewer complications and recover sooner,"[1] and she has developed a simple five-step program that can help anyone achieve these results. The book is a practical guide to using relaxation, visualization, healing affirmations, spiritual and emotional support, and meeting with your doctor in order to get the best results from surgery.

Huddleston's five steps are
1. Relax to feel peaceful
2. Visualize your healing
3. Organize a support group

4. Use healing statements
5. Meet your anesthesiologist

I didn't follow this program rigidly, but I did apply all these principles as I prepared for my surgery, especially the relaxation and visualization techniques. The book has an accompanying relaxation tape, but I preferred to use one by Elizabeth Crane of CTCA. I also created my own affirmations and added visualization techniques with which I was familiar. I affirmed and visualized that the operation would go well, with a good surgical outcome, a smooth recovery, and healing without any problems.

Bernie Siegel in *Love, Medicine, and Miracles* speaks of the important effects of positive affirmations and prayer. These techniques can reduce stress, normalize your pulse and blood pressure, and minimize the side effects of surgery. Relaxation reduces pain, which means that less pain-control medication is needed.

Bernie Siegel also speaks of the importance of what is said in the operating room while the patient is asleep under the anesthetic. I have always believed that patients hear what is said in the operating room, even if they do not remember the specifics of the conversations. The patient has a Higher Self that is not asleep during the operation. The patient also has a subconscious mind that takes it all in, and often the body will respond to what is happening.

There are many reports of patients recalling that they were floating above the operating table, observing their body being operated on but not feeling anything at all. Being aware of this kind of report and knowing about the Higher Self, when I was an anesthesiologist I would often talk to my patients while they were asleep during surgery.

I developed the habit of frequently putting a hand on their head to let them know that I was there with them. I would often speak gently in their ear to let them know that the operation was going well and to give them relevant information. I would tell them that they would wake up quietly and calmly without pain and with their organs functioning normally.

Depending on the area being operated on, I might give more specific instruction. For example, after surgery to the leg, I might say, "The blood supply in your leg will be very good, with good perfusion. Your leg will feel warm and comfortable and will look pink and healthy." In other cases I might affirm that their bladder and bowels would work normally after they recovered, even if problems in these areas were expected.

Nurses in the recovery room would often comment that they noticed a difference with my patients—they woke up quietly and in a calm and relaxed state. Nurses are very observant, and they told me that they could often tell whose patients were whose in the recovery room. At first I was skeptical, until one said, "Doctor ———'s patients always cry and are restless. Watch when his next one comes back from surgery." I waited and watched, and sure enough, she was right.

I wish that I had known about Bernie Siegel's work when I was practicing medicine, as I could have been even more effective in my work. Dr. Siegel would often give his patients very specific instructions. For example, if there was a problem with excessive bleeding, he would ask the patient to direct the blood away from the surgical site in order to reduce bleeding. He found that it worked. On one occasion, the pulse rate of a patient in surgery had gone up to 130. He told the patient, "You're doing well. Don't be nervous. I'd like your pulse to be 83." The patient's pulse came down to exactly 83 within a few minutes and stayed there.[2] I was thrilled when I first read that.

He recommends that patients ask their surgeon or anesthetist to read positive statements to them while under anesthetic. The patient can also recite these statements before surgery, and this was one purpose of the tapes to which I listened. I preferred to take the cassette player and headphones into surgery with me to be played while I was asleep, and my doctors were very willing to accommodate this request. If I were working in an operating room today, I would play gentle and soothing music, preferably classical, for the effect that it has on the body and the emotions. I would talk to my patients and have them work with me even while they were asleep.

TALK TO YOUR BODY

I talked to my body before anesthesia and let it know what was happening and what to expect. I have learned that just as plants and animals have guardian presences caring for them, so each of us has a guardian spirit that works with our body, helping to restore it to normal health and promoting healing after an event such as surgery. This little spirit is called the body elemental.[3] I told my body and body elemental exactly what was going to be done during surgery and what my desired outcome was. I was very specific and asked for good pain control, an easy waking from the anesthetic, no bleeding or infection postoperatively, fast and complete healing of the wound without undue scarring, and no ill effects or long-term problems. And it worked quite well.

I had seen my husband use this technique when he had surgery to remove two wisdom teeth. Anticipating that it might be a difficult operation, he prepared his body for several days. He told it that the teeth needed to go, and to "let go" of them ahead of time. The operation went smoothly with very little bleeding, and the teeth came out more easily than expected.

PRAYER

I asked friends to pray for me while I was under the anesthetic. I told them the name of the surgeon and asked them to pray specifically for him and the other hospital staff and for the best possible outcome. I asked them to visualize the room filled with light and healing energy and to ask for the Higher Selves of those involved to act at all times and to give direction as to the best course of action.

Under anesthesia you are not in control of your body, so it is nice to know that someone is specifically praying for you, or "holding the balance." I felt that I was in God's hands knowing that my husband was in the waiting room, praying for me and sending me positive healing energy. (I did the same for him when he had his dental surgery.)

I also prayed for myself ahead of the operation and commended myself to the protection of Archangel Michael and to angels of healing under the direction of Archangel Raphael and Mother Mary. I prayed for all in the operating room to be guided and overshadowed by the Holy Spirit. I asked for the angels and masters of healing to guide the hands of the surgeon and the anesthesiologist. I let the doctors know that people were praying for them, and they were happy to hear this.

I can truly say that I felt the presence of the angels, and I was not afraid. While I was in the recovery room waking up from the anesthetic, I heard "Pomp and Circumstance," by Elgar, the music that is associated with the master known as El Morya. I was surprised and very moved to hear this music, and I felt the tangible presence of the angels and the master when the music was playing. I wept, because I knew he was with me and that the biopsy of the lymph nodes would be negative. I do not know how I knew this—I just did. Of course, I could not prove anything, and I did not share this with anyone but my husband. I simply waited for the surgeon to give me the results the next day, and he confirmed that none of the eight lymph nodes had shown any sign of cancer.

HERBS AND SUPPLEMENTS

There are herbal remedies that may be helpful for faster healing and recovery. I used several different herbal teas, supplements, and lotions, preoperatively and postoperatively. These included pau d'arco tea, violet tea, oat straw tea, maitake mushroom extract, vitamin-E cream, Saint John's Wort oil, and the Arnica Montana homeopathic remedy. I checked all of this out with my surgeon first, as some herbal remedies can increase blood supply or reduce blood clotting, and hence increase bleeding during surgery.[4]

EXERCISE AND MASSAGE

Exercises are essential for postoperative recovery and are usually recommended for you by an occupational therapist. Gentle   walking and swimming are often helpful because they get the body moving, the lymph and the blood circulating, and the energy in the body flowing again without causing any unnecessary stress. Some fellow patients told me that they found yoga and tai chi to be calming and strengthening following surgery.

If you have undergone lymph-node surgery for breast cancer, gentle massage may be very helpful during recovery. The physical therapist with CTCA did wonderful work on the muscles of my arm, neck, shoulders, and back. I noticed an immediate improvement in my range of movement after these treatments.

I also used *Recovering from Breast Surgery: Exercises to Strengthen Your Body and Relieve Pain*, by Dianna Stumm. As well as providing specific exercises to help retain a full range of movement after surgery, she covers the very important subject of lymphedema, which is something to be aware of after lymph-node surgery. My surgeon had removed only eight of the lymph nodes under my arm, so it was very likely that I would not have any major problem after the surgical wound had healed. Even so, I was advised not to have blood drawn or blood pressure measured on my right arm (the side that received the surgery) for the rest of my life.

Rest

Finally, I was surprised at how tired I felt and how much sleep I needed postoperatively. I am sure that some of this was simply relief after a period of great stress. Nevertheless, any kind of surgery itself is a stress to the body. You may feel fine outwardly soon after the initial recovery period, but it often takes a lot longer to fully regain your inner strength and stamina. It is important to give yourself the needed time to rest and recover. Don't try to resume a full schedule too soon.

The Gift of Surgery

From a spiritual perspective, I understand that surgery and anesthesia are a great gift, and life would be far more difficult without them. Even as recently as a few hundred years ago, people suffered horribly from wounds on the battlefield or in day-to-day life. And if you believe in reincarnation, you could argue that we still carry the memory of this pain with us. Safe surgery and the ability to be asleep while you are operated on are tremendous blessings, ones that I pondered often when I put people to sleep for their surgery.

I was happy to have the cancer removed, as this would be one less thing for my body to deal with. It clearly had not been able to identify the cancer and deal with it by itself. With the tumor gone, the body now had a fresh start in dealing with the underlying causes that had allowed the cancer to form in the first place, without having to focus all its energy on dissolving the tumor.

There are times when surgery is exactly the right thing to do. If nothing else, it can buy time to make necessary changes at all levels, including strengthening the immune system so that it will better recognize cancer cells in the future.

CHECKLIST: PREPARING FOR SURGERY

✓ Know what to expect. Do your research and talk with your surgeon. Meet your anesthesiologist.

✓ Use relaxation techniques.

✓ Visualize a good outcome.

✓ Talk to your body. Tell it what to expect and let it know clearly what you would like it to do.

✓ Pray and ask others to pray for you.

✓ Use healing affirmations.

✓ Use herbs, supplements and other natural remedies to promote healing. (Check with your doctor first.)

✓ Exercise appropriately to speed recovery.

✓ Rest when you need it. Don't try to resume a full schedule too soon.

CHAPTER 8

AN INTEGRATED APPROACH
TO HEALING

The all-or-nothing approach has never appealed to me—only traditional or only alternative, and never the twain shall meet. In my medical practice, I have seen the benefit of both, and I have learned that very few things in life are absolute.

Having worked in trauma centers and emergency rooms, I can wholeheartedly agree with Dr. Andrew Weil, when he said, "If I'm involved in a serious auto accident, I want the ambulance to take me to the nearest high-tech trauma center. Mainstream medicine is definitely the way to go for serious injuries." There are times when surgery, antibiotics, and modern medicine are truly lifesaving.

Dr. Weil continues, "But let's say I developed chronic pain as a result of the accident. Beyond narcotics, mainstream medicine doesn't have much to offer. But several complementary therapies can help. I might try chiropractic, acupuncture, yoga, massage, or visualization therapy."[1] There are times when natural methods, such as homeopathy, acupuncture, and naturopathy, work better than anything else. I like to use the term complementary instead of alternative when talking about these therapies, since it implies these other healing arts are working together with conventional treatments.

In my own life, I combine the two. Here is one example: I often travel overseas to conduct seminars, and I always take with me a small array of pharmaceutical and complementary remedies to cover the kinds of illnesses that can burden the weary traveler. CranActin, a concentrated extract of cranberry juice, is one of the items in my kit. Cranberry juice is a well-known remedy for bladder and urinary-tract infections, and the concentrated extract in a capsule is much easier to carry than a large bottle of juice. I have used it as a preventative or at the earliest sign of an infection, and it is usually very effective.[2]

If traveling overseas I also carry a course of antibiotics, and although I have rarely had to use them, I have been very glad to have them when CranActin did not do the trick. I do not hesitate to take antibiotics when I need to—which, fortunately, has been infrequently—while at the same time treating by natural means the yeast infection that sometimes results from the antibiotics.

Although I have been comfortable for many years blending complementary and traditional medicines, particularly in treating less serious forms of illness, it was a different challenge to blend the two to treat cancer—a challenge I had never thought I would have to face.

CHOOSING A PRACTITIONER

I have good friends who are naturopaths, chiropractors and alternative health care practitioners in Australia and in the United States, and I respect their work. I have referred people to them from my medical practice. These practitioners also respect the medical profession and, more importantly, know when to refer someone who needs standard medical care. This is a key point to consider when you are choosing an alternative healthcare professional.

I vividly remember ending a friendship with one naturopath in Australia. I got to know her socially, and she expressed a desire to consult with me about some of her cases. I was cautious, but agreed to see how a working relationship might evolve. It did not last long. Soon after our conversation, she left a series of messages on my answering machine at home. I was out at the time and did not receive them until arriving home much later.

A worried couple had brought their young child to her practice, and she thought the illness sounded like meningitis (which is life-threatening). Instead of sending the parents to the emergency room immediately, she tried several homeopathic remedies. They were not my patients, but she called me to seek my advice and reassurance.

As I listened to her messages, one after another, I became more and more alarmed. I called back immediately and found that the parents, thankfully, had wearied of the situation and taken their child to the emergency room at the children's hospital. Fortunately, a lumbar puncture to sample the spinal fluid showed that the child did not have meningitis. The doctors determined it was a viral infection that would clear up within a few days.

I immediately invited the naturopath over to my home and tried to get an understanding of her thinking. I thought that perhaps she did not understand the implications of meningitis and how time is of the essence in order to prevent death or permanent damage to the central nervous system. However, as we spoke it became clear that she did understand these things, but had wanted to see how her homeopathics would work. I shared my utter dismay that she would be willing to risk the life of a child to satisfy her curiosity.

She then shared a couple of other case histories that alarmed me even further. I again pointed out the risks she was taking, but she could not see my point of view at all. She simply "wanted to see if the remedies would work." I was left feeling that I had just interviewed one of the people that M. Scott Peck speaks of in his book *People of the Lie,* who seem to be incapable of feeling compassion or empathy for other people and seem to be only concerned about themselves. After recognizing this behavior, I came to the conclusion that she was dangerous and I could no longer continue the relationship.

I know that she is not representative of the many capable healthcare professionals in the field of complementary medicine and the healing arts. I could also give you examples of medical doctors that I knew who were appallingly negligent in their behavior. I merely present this as an experience that has helped shape my life, personally and professionally.

EVALUATING DIFFERENT THERAPIES

As I approached the treatment of my breast cancer, I fully believed that it was possible to combine the best of traditional and complementary medicine to develop the best possible program for me. I believe that all of us can do the same, and it seems that many cancer patients agree. Some surveys have found that more than 80 percent of breast-cancer patients use some form of complementary medicine in addition to their traditional health care—even though many of them do not tell their doctors.

Initially, as I delved into the choices in alternative cancer treatment, I found them to be absolutely bewildering. You cannot imagine the variety of choices until you have cancer. Suddenly, you see articles and books everywhere about this or that alternative treatment for cancer. And once you order a supplement or vitamin or herb, all kinds of unsolicited material starts arriving in the mailbox. A lot of it can seem downright flaky or weird, or at best unsubstantiated. I especially disliked the ones that claimed outright that they "cure cancer." I felt that I could dismiss them right away. Or could I? I read everything that came into my hands just in case there was something out there that might provide a clue to my best treatment.

What I found is probably what you would expect. Much of the evidence supporting alternative treatments is anecdotal. There are very few studies, double-blind trials or other means of scientifically evaluating them. This was very frustrating for the doctor in me. Everyone seems to know someone who tried this or that herb or treatment and "it worked." However, all that really means is that it worked for them, for their condition, at that time. It does not necessarily mean that it will work for me and for what I have. And what else were they doing at the same time that was also a part—and perhaps the real cause—of their healing?

I quickly realized that at some time or another, almost any "cure" or "curative agent," even the most unlikely, had probably cured at least someone of some kind of cancer. But one case was not enough for me—unless, of course, I was that one case! This only goes to show the uniqueness of cancer, or perhaps, more importantly, of the people who contract it.

The patient in me was willing to try almost anything, as long as there was a chance it might work. The doctor in me was more cautious. Fortunately, the minister in me often came to the rescue to integrate the two. How was I to know whether or not a particular treatment was likely to work? In many cases, I didn't have the solid proof I would have liked to see, but somehow I had to navigate through it all. And I certainly wanted to look at and evaluate the options without spending a fortune!

Fortunately, scientific research has been done in recent years about many complementary therapies, and there is a lot more solid information about what really works and what does not than existed ten or twenty years ago. I found several books by authors who had done the hard work of compiling this research, and this was a good starting point for my own evaluations. (I have included information about these books and some more recent ones in the resources section at the end of this chapter.)

I also approached my healing with a spiritual principle taught to me by my teacher: all healing occurs through the direction of the Higher Self and through the light.* All methods of healing, whatever their source, are simply modes of delivering light to stimulate or allow the body to heal itself. This explains why one person may need surgery and traditional treatment, another can be healed by prayer alone, while yet another can use herbs and get fantastic results. Everyone is different, and each person needs a different quality of light to bring their body and their being to a

---

* I use the word *light* here to indicate spiritual energy, the essence that originates from the heart of creation. This energy has many names and manifestations. It is often seen by mystics and clairvoyants as "light."

point of balance and healing.

My approach was to read widely and research as much as possible. I think that I can now honestly say that I have heard of or read about almost every possible treatment method or modality for breast cancer. I never dismissed anything out of hand until I had read about it and weighed it in my heart.

MAKING CHOICES

About three weeks after my diagnosis, I was still examining my options and eventually made what I felt were heartfelt and centered decisions. Making these choices did not mean that I was fixed in my approach, but it did help me feel that I was developing my own treatment plan. If I needed to adjust it as I went along, that was fine too.

It was becoming more and more clear that I needed to go through with chemotherapy and radiation, as I did not want to leave my treatment solely to complementary therapies. I had seen too many friends and patients with cancer do poorly with complementary therapies alone.

Having decided that I would combine conventional and complementary therapies, I began to look for ways to boost my immune system to help me to fight the cancer and to reduce the potential side effects of the conventional therapies. I knew chemotherapy would be a big challenge to my body, and I felt as if I was in training for a marathon that would require intense preparation; I would need to dig deeply within myself and into my energy reserves.

I also wanted to get to the cause and core of the condition of cancer, if possible, and eliminate it so the cancer would not return. Along the way, if I stumbled across the miracle cure, that would be all well and good. However, I was not about to put all my eggs in one basket.

One of the reasons I decided to have my treatment at Cancer Treatment Centers of America is because their staff were aware of the benefits of complementary therapies. They encourage their patients to use them, and they incorporate a number of these therapies into the program at their hospitals. They seek to treat the whole person.

I had not seen anywhere else such a complete program of state-of-the-art traditional medical techniques combined with complementary therapies, and I felt that they would understand my approach and would be able to provide a framework that I could not find anywhere else.

An integrated approach to cancer treatment is becoming more popular, and there are a number of cancer centers that integrate complementary therapies with medical care. More doctors are becoming aware of the benefits of complementary therapies and are supportive of them, even when these therapies are not part of the formal programs at their centers.

The more I read, the more my feelings were confirmed that no single treatment or therapy would do the job for me. And since cancer is not just an illness affecting a single organ—it is a condition that affects the whole body, the whole organism—the approach I took would also need to address every area of my being. It would need to be holistic.

It was becoming clear that I would need to include elements of the following therapies in my treatment program:

1. Nutrition, diet, and dietary supplements
2. Exercise and movement
3. Other complementary therapies, including herbs, naturopathy, homeopathy, and Chinese medicine (acupuncture and Chinese herbs)
4. Lifestyle changes to reduce my risk factors and support my immune system
5. Work with the mind-body connection and forms of stress reduction, including meditation and music therapy
6. Counseling and work on relationships
7. Spiritual support

These were the choices I made, and I am fully aware that they are only mine. I knew myself and had to follow my heart. You may have different circumstances, and you might not make these same choices even in circumstances similar to mine. You know yourself best and what will work for you.

I believe that people have an inner sense about what is right for them. I remember vividly one woman with advanced metastatic disease whom I met while I was being treated. She had begged her doctors to remove both breasts when the cancer was first diagnosed, but they would not. She said that she knew in her heart that she would also get cancer in the second breast, and she was right. Now here she was with secondaries in her brain and bones. Her doctors eventually performed bilateral mastectomies, but it was too late. She passed on shortly thereafter, greatly saddened not to be able to see her young son grow up. It was a hard thing to listen to her story and to meet her family. It left an important impression on me and other cancer patients who met her. We really do know ourselves best, and our courses are individual.

I was now becoming interested in remedies and treatments that I almost felt were drawing me to them. It was as if I was being led to what felt right to me. Other patients have described the same phenomenon. There is a sense of rightness about what you are doing. Even if at the time you may not be sure of the way to go, in retrospect your choices will prove to be right. In my case, I felt greatly supported by the prayers and spiritual work that I was doing and that others were doing on my behalf. I believe that they made a huge difference and helped me make the right choices.

In the following chapters, I will describe the different complementary therapies that I chose and explain a little about why I made those choices and how I incorporated these therapies into my treatment plan.

RESOURCES FOR RESEARCH ON ALTERNATIVE AND COMPLEMENTARY CANCER THERAPIES

There is not room in this book to include a comprehensive evaluation of all the complementary and alternative cancer therapies that are available. However, here are a few books that provide this information. Get the latest edition to make sure you have the most up-to-date data and research results.

Cancer: Increasing Your Odds for Survival: A Resource Guide for Integrating Mainstream, Alternative, and Complementary Therapies
DAVID BOGNAR

When I was first diagnosed with breast cancer, a friend who was recovering from her own gynecological surgery found this book in the hospital bookstore and sent it to me. It is a complete resource of cancer centers, treatment programs, and their options, along with pros and cons. Written by a man whose partner struggled with breast cancer, it is well-researched and gives an excellent overview of cancer, including detailed information on conventional, alternative and complementary, and supplemental treatments.

The book provides a balanced perspective, including sections on mind-body therapies, psychological aspects of cancer, and cancer and spirituality. This is a resource guide to help you to begin thinking about how to integrate mainstream and complementary therapies. I read it from cover the cover, and it confirmed many of my own intuitions.

One of the most useful aspects of the book is the information on success rates of different therapies. Even though there is often not enough clinical evidence to prove without a doubt whether a particular therapy is effective, Bognar provides an objective analysis of what evidence there is. I found myself returning again and again to this book as I looked at my choices.

This book has also been made into a four-hour documentary of the same name, hosted by Walter Cronkite. The videos are interesting and helpful, but the book contains more detail.

Breast Cancer: What You Should Know (But May Not Be Told) About Prevention, Diagnosis, and Treatment
STEVE AUSTIN AND CATHY HITCHCOCK

This book was written by a naturopath and his wife, a counselor and breast-cancer survivor. It gives a comprehensive analysis of the risks and benefits of conventional treatment options (surgery, radiation, and chemotherapy) and of several alternative and complementary therapies. Cathy tells the story of her experience with breast cancer and explains why she chose the treatment options she did. Even though your choices may be different, you will probably find her approach to the issues interesting and helpful.

Blended Medicine: How to Integrate the Best Mainstream and Alternative Remedies for Maximum Health and Healing
MICHAEL CASTLEMAN

Michael Castleman is a medical journalist and one of the top health writers in the country. He has written about mainstream medicine and complementary therapies for many years and has authored nine other books, including *Nature's Cures* and *The Healing Herbs.* He has worked with doctors and specialists in many areas.

Blended Medicine helps you look at the most effective treatment options from all disciplines and describes how to use them together to treat many common health problems. There is a section on cancer, which includes a practical guide to the different kinds of therapies and a summary of each. The book is easy to read. I recommend it for its balanced approach.

> *How to Prevent and Treat Cancer with Natural Medicine*
> MICHAEL T. MURRAY, TIM BIRDSALL, JOSEPH E. PIZZORNO, PAUL REILLY

This book provides a comprehensive survey of complementary therapies and their use in cancer treatment, both for fighting the cancer itself and to help with side effects of chemotherapy and radiation. Tim Birdsall is a naturopath at CTCA. The book is well researched and documented, citing numerous medical studies on the effectiveness (or not) of different treatments.

> *A Patient's Guide to Cancer Care*
> VIRGINIA B. MORRIS AND SOPHIE FORRESTER

This compact booklet provides a useful overview of every aspect of cancer, from diagnosis to conventional and complementary therapies to financial considerations. It also includes a list of resources.

CHECKLIST: BLENDING COMPLEMENTARY AND CONVENTIONAL MEDICINE

✓ **Choose medical practitioners who are open to complementary therapies.**

✓ **Choose complementary therapy practitioners who are also open to conventional therapies.**

✓ **Let all your practitioners know about all of your therapies** so they can avoid possible negative interactions.

✓ **Evaluate alternative treatments objectively.** Be open to your intuition as well.

✓ **Be selective.** You can't do every complementary therapy.

✓ **Consider the following options:**

   ○ Nutrition, diet, and dietary supplements

   ○ Exercise and movement

   ○ Herbs, naturopathy, homeopathy, Chinese medicine, and other complementary therapies

   ○ Lifestyle changes to reduce risk factors and support your immune system

   ○ Mind-body work and stress reduction, including meditation, music therapy, and visualization

   ○ Counseling and work on relationships

   ○ Spiritual support

Chapter 9

NUTRITION AND DIET

The National Cancer Institute tells us that one-third of all cancer deaths are related to malnutrition.[1] This is partly due to the disease itself interfering with digestion and assimilation of food, but in addition, cancer treatments themselves may result in decreased appetite, lower food intake, and impaired digestion, which lead to weight loss and depletion of nutrients in the body.

If you are undergoing cancer treatment, food is an essential weapon in the fight: it provides the energy, nutrients, and antioxidants the body needs for recovery and to fight the disease. Beyond this, there are many studies showing significant statistical correlations between diet and the incidence of cancer. If nutrition and diet can have such a profound effect on the onset of the disease, it makes sense to have diet be part of the treatment program.

I believe diet and nutrition are an essential subject when you are dealing with any cancer—both as an element in healing the body and in preventing recurrence.

You Really Are What You Eat

Unfortunately, I had been ignoring my diet for some time before I got cancer, and I believe that I paid a big price. How did a doctor who is interested in alternative healing and spiritual subjects get to be this way? It wasn't easy!

I had been brought up from late childhood with a fairly healthy, natural diet. My parents started seeking a better way to eat when my father was diagnosed with a stomach ulcer. He changed his diet and cured himself. Our family went through a phase of being mostly vegetarian and eating lots of fresh fruit and vegetables. Later we added fish, chicken, and other proteins.

Perhaps it was because I had been raised on a healthy diet that I never really appreciated it as much as I should have. I did not consciously decide to eat a less healthy diet, but it gradually happened that I was eating more processed foods, more sugar, more dairy products, and fewer vegetables. In fact, by the time I was diagnosed with breast cancer, I was not eating well at all. An increasingly stressful and busy lifestyle meant that I did not take time to look after myself in many areas of my life, diet being just one of them.

Food is an essential weapon in the fight against cancer.

After my diagnosis, my secretary told me that in the previous year, I mostly ate on the run: crackers and a cup of soup or instant noodles. I used to skip meals and fill in with bread or snacks that I could take to meetings. And I drank a lot of coffee—sometimes as many as eight or nine cups a day.

At first I was quite surprised when she told me this. I used to eat a couple of healthy meals a week, and somehow this was all I remembered. I still thought that I was eating reasonably well. It's amazing how we can fool ourselves when it comes to something as important as nutrition.

When I was diagnosed, I asked myself why I couldn't see it coming. As I look back now, particularly in the area of diet, I can see I was on a collision course.

Cancer is a great motivator! I now had a very good reason to eat well. Candace Vann, a friend and nutritionist, helped me develop a healthy meal plan that suited my needs, my appetite, and my taste buds.

I cut out most dairy foods, all forms of refined sugar, and all highly processed foods. I began to shop for organic fruits and vegetables whenever possible and increased my protein intake in the form of fish, organic chicken and turkey, soy, and other vegetable proteins. When I was hungry between meals, I had formed the habit of reaching for breads and other "filler" foods. I now disciplined myself to substitute something that would support my healing, such as raw or lightly steamed vegetables, which only took a few extra minutes to prepare.

When I made these changes to my diet and began taking the time to cook and prepare healthy food, I noticed, after several months, a big improvement in my overall well-being. My energy level increased, my complexion, skin texture, and skin tone improved, and my weight and digestion returned to normal. A number of other minor health problems cleared up as well. People kept commenting, "You look great" or "You look really well," even in the midst of chemotherapy. And I could start to see the effects myself in the mirror.

FOOD AS ENERGY

The energy in all the food we eat originally comes from the sun. Plants, through photosynthesis, use the energy of sunlight to grow. Animals eat the plants and convert that energy into a different form. All food, ultimately, is condensed sunlight, a way to take in the energy of the sun in a form that we can assimilate and use.

I believe that the food we eat also carries spiritual light, and the quality of this light varies in different types of food. Food is a means of delivering light to our bodies in a form that we can readily assimilate, and by choosing our food wisely, we can deliver to our bodies a specific quality of light that can assist in healing.

I knew that my body would need the physical energy of certain foods, as well as the light in those foods, in order to support the healing process. And I felt that my body would know what it needed. So instead of ignoring my body, I started to listen to it, and as I listened, I found that I began to crave some things more than others. For example, I began to crave the sea vegetables and pickled ginger that I had eaten some years before when I was on a macrobiotic diet.

When I talked about these cravings with Candace, I was interested to see how much my own body had been telling me what was correct for me to eat. Sea vegetables and ginger are rich in minerals and are known to help remove toxins from the body and stimulate the function of the liver, two things I needed to do during cancer treatment. Ginger is also used in treating the nausea associated with chemotherapy.

I also took a greater interest in the spiritual aspect of food and its preparation. I had known about this before but had been simply too busy to put it into practice. Now I had the time and the inclination, and I began to understand more fully the concept of healthy food as a medicine in itself. I returned to my old habit of blessing my food and giving thanks for it, asking for it to be charged with light and energy for my healing. I began to enjoy taking the time to prepare and eat my meals—it became a time of meditation and contemplation.

DIET AND CANCER

At CTCA I met their director of nutrition, Dr. Patrick Quillin, an expert in the field of cancer and nutrition and the author of the best-selling book *Beating Cancer with Nutrition*. In an article titled "The Breast Cancer/Nutrition Connection," Dr. Quillin says, "Cancer is a whole body disease, not just a regionalized lump or bump. We need to rethink our paradigm on treating breast cancer.... Nourishing the body's natural defenses can cut cancer risk by up to 90 percent. A healthy diet can encourage the immune system to recognize and destroy cancer before it becomes a palpable lump."[2] In the article, he draws attention to several key areas that still motivate my choice of foods today.

~

NOURISHING THE BODY'S NATURAL DEFENSES CAN CUT CANCER RISK BY UP TO 90 PERCENT.
—Dr. Patrick Quillin

Fat in the Diet
"People, such as the Japanese, Seventh Day Adventists, and Mormons, who eat a low-fat diet have one-half to one-fifth the breast cancer incidence of the normal American. Cut fat intake from 40 percent of calories down to a healthier 20 percent of calories by eating less beef, dairy foods, margarine, and fried foods."[3]

There is a lot of scientific and statistical evidence that you can significantly decrease your risk for breast cancer if you use healthier oils, such as olive oil or flaxseed oil, in place of the saturated fats and hydrogenated and heavily-processed oils that are most often found in supermarkets today.

The alpha linolenic acid in flaxseed oil has been shown to have suppressive effects on breast cancer cells. My naturopath says that this makes sense especially for the estrogen-sensitive cancers. It theoretically binds to the estrogen receptors and decreases the proliferation of estrogen-sensitive breast cancer cells. Flaxseed oil is relatively inexpensive and can be easily added to the diet.

Olive oil is a staple in the diet of Mediterranean countries, and its use is linked statistically to lower breast cancer rates. Extra virgin olive oil is the healthiest type of olive oil and is widely available in supermarkets. While the use of polyunsaturated vegetable oils has been shown to reduce the incidence of heart disease, many of these oils actually increase the risk of breast cancer. Olive oil, however, has proven beneficial in reducing the risk for both heart disease and breast cancer.[4]

Omega-3 fish oils are an essential part of any anti-cancer diet. Studies have shown a reduced cancer risk—particularly for breast cancer—in those who take fish oil in their diet. Taken in capsule form, it is tasteless and easy to digest. Fish oil supplements lower blood pressure and triglycerides and improve heart health. They are also believed to reduce inflammation, which may play a role in some cancers as well as heart disease.

Sugar in the Diet

"Of twenty-one countries studied, the average sugar intake in that country dictates the breast cancer incidence. Avoid white sugar and its many cousins: corn syrup, dextrose, sucrose. Cut your intake of all sweets by 75 percent."[5]

Many people feel they need a certain amount of sweetness in their diet for a sense of balance. You can often reduce your need for sweet foods by cutting down on salt and meat in the diet. If you do need sweet foods, the best sources are the natural sweetness of fresh fruits and vegetables and their juices. These sources also provide an abundance of vitamins and minerals that your body needs.

Antioxidants

On a cellular level, a primary cause of cancer is free radicals, which attack the DNA and cell membrane. Antioxidants counter the effects of oxidation and protect the body on a cellular level from the effects of free radicals and many environmental pollutants. They also strengthen the immune system and help it to fight the cancer more effectively.

Many fruits and vegetables are high in antioxidants. In general, look for foods that are higher in color: red grapes rather than white, sweet potatoes rather than white potatoes, spinach rather than lettuce.

SOY PRODUCTS

Breast cancer is known as a "hormonally driven" cancer. The body's hormones, particularly estrogen, stimulate the growth and development of breast cancer cells. Recently, there has been a lot of interest in the use of soy as a breast cancer preventative. Soybeans contain a substance called genistein, which interacts with estrogen receptors in the body.

Dr. Bob Arnot, author of *The Breast Cancer Prevention Diet*, says, "Premenopausal Chinese women have about a 50 percent decrease in breast cancer risk when they consume high amounts of soy.... A case-control study from Australia showed a significant reduction in pre- and postmenopausal breast cancer for those women eating high amounts of soy and other foods containing weak estrogens. That's also been observed in America in vegetarian women with high soy intakes, who also have lower risks of breast cancer."[6] Dr. Arnot's book confirms what many are now saying: that nutrition is emerging as one of the most important ways to prevent breast cancer. His book includes a comprehensive study of the use of soy in a breast-cancer-prevention diet.

However, before adding soy to the diet, a breast-cancer patient should first check whether their particular type of cancer is estrogen-sensitive. Studies in test tubes and with animals have shown that genistein stimulates the growth of estrogen-receptor-positive cancers. It is not yet known whether this finding will carry over to humans or not, but until further research is done, it makes sense for women with estrogen-receptor-positive breast cancer to restrict soy intake (no more than four servings per week) and not take soy supplements.[7]

If you plan to include soy in your program, soy milk is a good substitute for regular milk and an easy way to add soy to the diet. Different brands use different recipes and often taste quite different. Keep trying until you find one you like. Tofu is another good source for soy. Try various brands and alternate methods of preparation. Asian and macrobiotic cookbooks have recipes for tasty and satisfying meals using tofu.

THE MACROBIOTIC DIET

Some years before I developed breast cancer, I had been on a more-or-less macrobiotic diet for some time. I had heard claims about the macrobiotic diet being able to "cure" cancer and had read of people who claimed to have cured themselves in this way. I also had a friend with metastatic melanoma, a cancer that is nearly always fatal, who attributed her still being alive fifteen years later to a strict macrobiotic diet. Therefore, when I was diagnosed, I definitely wanted to find out more about the macrobiotic diet and what it could do for me.

What I found is that many elements of the macrobiotic diet make sense according to the best scientific research into cancer and nutrition. It is low in fat and high in fiber, uses whole grains, avoids red meat, and includes fish, soy protein, and lots of vegetables. All of these things will be helpful, no matter what diet you choose.

I was not able to find any scientific studies to show that the macrobiotic diet in itself can cure cancer. However, I did find one study of late-stage prostate cancer patients that showed that those on a macrobiotic diet lived an average of 177 months, compared to 91 months in the control group.[8] Other evidence seemed to point to the same conclusion: that a macrobiotic diet could extend the life of someone with cancer but was not a cure in itself. However, even this is very significant, and no doubt the people in this study were very grateful for the average of seven years extra that they lived.

My conclusion was that the principles of the macrobiotic diet would be helpful in putting together my plan. Many of the recommendations I had already decided to follow were part of the diet, and people who had been working with the diet for many years had evolved a way of incorporating these principles into appealing and satisfying meals. It felt good to me.

I did not follow a strict macrobiotic diet but made adaptations according to what the scientific evidence showed, as well as what I felt my body was telling me I needed.

If you feel called to pursue a more rigorous macrobiotic diet as part of your healing program, I would recommend getting advice from someone with expertise so as to avoid potential pitfalls (such as B-12 deficiency) that some people have run into when they tried to follow it strictly without the necessary understanding and experience.

WATCH YOUR WEIGHT

Fats can oxidize to form free radicals. Fat cells also produce estrogen, which stimulates the growth of breast cancer. Excess weight also increases the risk of cancer of the colon, kidney, esophagus and uterus. Therefore, if you are dealing with breast cancer or any type of cancer, or simply want to prevent cancer, try to maintain your optimum weight, or at least decrease your weight if you are overweight.[9]

VITAMINS AND SUPPLEMENTS

I was never one for handfuls of supplements, as I always thought that I would get all the nutrients I needed if I "ate well" and maintained a "balanced diet." Sadly, this is often not the case today. In the last fifty years or so there has been a marked decline in the quality of foods that we eat and a decrease in the amount of nutrients in these foods. This is especially important to consider if you are dealing with cancer and its treatment, which create big demands on the immune system.

In addition to improving my diet and the quality of food, I began to take supplements and vitamins, some recommended by the nutritionists at CTCA and others added based on my own research. I didn't go overboard, but I tried to be sensible. I attribute some of my improved health and well-being to the vitamins and supplements I took. It is important to remember that the taking of supplements is not a substitute for eating correctly each day.

When you are dealing with a more-than-ordinary stress on the immune system (like cancer or cancer therapies), supplemental antioxidants are recommended. A good daily program would include 1,000 mg of vitamin C, 25,000 IU of beta-carotene, 400 IU of vitamin E, a good multi-vitamin, and 200 mcg of selenium.* Many cancer patients take additional antioxidants such as coenzyme Q-10, grapeseed extract, and glutathione.

Especially important for cancer treatment and prevention is vitamin D. It acts in the body as both a vitamin and a hormone and is most commonly known for its key role in calcium absorption and the prevention of osteoporosis. More recently it is coming into prominence in cancer treatment, as a result of the many studies that have shown a correlation between low levels of this vitamin and higher incidence of many types of cancer.[10] It is now commonly prescribed in cancer prevention and for those who are dealing with cancer, usually at a dose of 400 to 1,000 IU per day. Some oncologists and naturopaths recommend higher doses adjusted according to tests of serum levels.

My Diet Today

These days my diet is not as strict as it was while I was in treatment, but I still consider nutrition a part of my daily fight against the return of cancer. I try to remember that it took a long time for me to develop the cancer and that many seemingly insignificant daily choices made up the sum total of my life and this outcome.

I put an emphasis on organic whole foods and plenty of fresh vegetables. Fish is a primary source of protein and omega-3 fatty acids. I also eat eggs and poultry (free range and chemical free, if available) and vegetarian proteins in the form of soy and gluten products. I occasionally have meat or dairy products. I minimize sugar and refined foods, and I read the labels when I buy food, looking for natural and organic ingredients. It takes a bit more time and some discipline, but I

---

* Selenium in excess can be harmful. Since many multivitamin and antioxidant supplements also contain selenium, be sure to include the amounts in these products when calculating your total daily dose. Don't exceed 200 mcg from all sources combined.

think the results are worthwhile.

Having said all that, I think that I am balanced about nutrition. I enjoy food and eating well, and if I come to eat at your home, I usually enjoy whatever you put in front of me. If I want an occasional treat, I will indulge myself. In general, I am more aware of what I eat, and I am making better choices.

I feel that the changes in diet helped greatly in my healing. As an added benefit, I think the changed diet also helped to minimize the effects of menopause, which was brought on by the chemotherapy agents.

I notice that when I stray from a healthy diet for any length of time that it affects me in so many ways—physically, mentally, and emotionally. When I dealt with the local recurrence after years of being cancer-free, I had strayed from my diet and cut back on the supplements and antioxidants. I quickly corrected my course.

PUTTING TOGETHER YOUR PLAN

Diet is very personal and individual. What works for one person may not work for another, yet the basic principles of a healthy diet do apply to everyone.

When you are deciding on what diet you will follow, it is important to listen to what your body is telling you. Your body is designed to work with natural, whole foods, and if you can cut down on artificial and processed foods, you give it the best opportunity to send you clearer signals about what it needs.

For example, if you find yourself craving sweets, it is probably not because your body needs refined sugar. It may be that it needs vitamin C, potassium, and other nutrients that are found in nature in conjunction with the sweet tastes that come primarily from fruits. Sodas and artificial sweeteners don't have these nutrients, therefore they don't meet the underlying needs the body is expressing, and using them may lead to an intensification of the craving.

Some cancer patients do very well without changing their diet.

However, many feel that a change in diet is beneficial, and science is beginning to clearly support this. You may find it helpful to talk to a nutritionist, especially one who is experienced in diet for cancer patients. This is especially important if you are thinking of making major changes in your diet. A good nutritionist can help you interpret the messages your body is sending you, sort through a lot of information, prioritize, and put together a practical, balanced program.

Eat food that you enjoy, and perhaps learn to enjoy different foods than you have before.

CHECKLIST: A CANCER-FIGHTING DIET

✓ Cut down on dairy foods and red meats, refined sugars, and all highly processed foods.

✓ Use healthier oils such as olive oil and flaxseed.

✓ Increase vegetables and fruits, especially the brightly colored ones, which provide cancer fighting antioxidants to boost the immune system.

✓ Supplement with vitamins and antioxidants, including 1,000 mg of vitamin C, 25,000 IU of beta-carotene, Omega-3 fish oil, 400 to 1,000 IU of vitamin D, 400 IU of vitamin E, a good multivitamin, and 200 mcg of selenium. Additional antioxidants such as coenzyme Q-10, grapeseed extract, and glutathione can also help.

✓ Work to maintain your optimum weight.

✓ Find what works for you. Get some expert help from a nutritionist to customize your own program.

CHAPTER 10

EXERCISE FOR INCREASED VITALITY

D r. Linn Goldberg, author of *Exercise for Prevention and Treatment of Illness* and an expert on the use of exercise in healing, has said, "If the effects of exercise could be bottled, it would be the most widely prescribed medication."[1]

Exercise is especially important for breast cancer prevention. Nutritionist and cancer expert Dr. Patrick Quillin says, "Exercise is one of the cheapest, easiest, most nontoxic and effective ways a woman can beat the odds on breast cancer. Walk, bike, stair step, do aerobics, horseback ride, rollerblade. Work with your healthcare professional to determine your abilities and limitations."[2]

I must admit I had never been much for exercise. I led a sedentary lifestyle, especially at work, where a lot of time was spent on the phone, at a computer, or in meetings. Even after work, my preference for recreation was to lay on the couch with a good book. Occasionally I would take a twenty-minute walk with Peter—if he really encouraged me.

I knew I was not fit, but I didn't realize how unfit I was until a month before my diagnosis. We were visiting Peter's family in Sydney, Australia, and we had all walked down to the harbor to watch the fireworks on New Year's Eve. I was fine on the way there, which was downhill. But on the way back I had to pause and catch my breath frequently. There was no way I could even keep up with Peter's mother, who was nearly seventy. I remember remarking to her that she was fitter than I was and did not seem to have any problem with the hills. She told me later that she was worried about me.

I really became alarmed after my diagnosis, when I read the statistics about cancer and exercise. I already knew that exercise helped prevent cardiovascular disease and that it promoted general good health. But I was surprised to find that physical activity or exercise can cut overall cancer risk nearly in half. The greater the level of activity, the lower the risk, especially in colon and breast cancers.[3]

Reading these statistics, I knew I had to reassess my lifestyle. I realized anew that exercise is not just something that is nice to do for active people. It is simply part of what it takes to make it in the modern world.

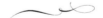

IF THE EFFECTS OF EXERCISE COULD BE BOTTLED,

IT WOULD BE THE MOST WIDELY PRESCRIBED MEDICATION.
—Dr. Linn Goldberg

From a physical perspective, there are many benefits. Regular moderate exercise for about thirty minutes per day or even every second day boosts your immune system. It helps normalize body weight and get rid of excess fat, a known risk factor in breast cancer. Exercise gets the blood and lymph fluid circulating and helps the body get rid of toxins.[4]

Exercise also lifts your spirits and helps with depression and anxiety, which many people deal with after a diagnosis of cancer. And just as exercise clears the cobwebs in the mind and the body, it also helps to clear them spiritually. Exercise is a way to enhance the flow of light in the body and to increase the body's vitality.

Here was another wake-up call, another area of life where I would have to make changes. Inspired by what I had read, I started walking for thirty minutes a day. We live in a rural subdivision overlooking the Yellowstone River. The snow-covered Absaroka Range rises to twelve thousand feet on the other side of the valley. I slowed down my mind and took in the sights, the beautiful mountains, the flowers by the roadside, the Yellowstone River as it winds its way through the Paradise Valley, the clouds as they move through the sky. It was all very beautiful, and I was amazed to realize that although I had walked here many times before, I had never really seen the view—I was always thinking about problems at work or the next thing that needed to be done.

Now I saw it all through new eyes. As I walked, I played inspirational music on headphones, listened to tapes on the subject of healing, or recited the rosary. I invariably arrived back home energized and uplifted. I remain motivated to continue this daily practice and use a treadmill in winter.

PHYSICAL ACTIVITY OR EXERCISE CAN CUT OVERALL

CANCER RISK NEARLY IN HALF.

As a doctor, I had often told my patients to get regular exercise. But my job had been to deal with the other aspects of their treatment, and exercise was not something I stressed, and I really did not pay attention to it for myself. It was therefore helpful to have some assistance in putting together a program. During chemotherapy and radiation, I worked with Colleen, a physical therapist who held classes at the hospital and had developed a series of stretching and strengthening exercises for cancer patients. The exercises were simple and easy to do, yet effective. Colleen encouraged me to be realistic, to start slowly and not to overdo it. She also explained that even a little exercise each day or every other day is *much* better than doing nothing.

What surprised me the most was how much exercise helped with the side effects of chemotherapy. During chemo I did not feel like exercising precisely because I was not feeling good. And with a lot of other things on my mind, it seemed that exercise was the last thing to be worried about. But when I pushed myself to do some physical activity, it really helped. It got me out of the chair and got the circulation going. Even in small amounts, it definitely helped with the side effects of nausea, tiredness and lethargy. It also provided a welcome distraction and a different perspective on life. Towards the end of my chemotherapy sessions, I was doing daily laps around the nurses' station with my IV pole and chemo pump in tow.

When I was able to, I combined Colleen's simple daily program with aerobic walking. Within two weeks of starting the program I noticed an even greater improvement in my energy level as well as greater flexibility.

During my six weeks of radiation therapy, a group of patients got together each day for thirty minutes to do the recommended exercises. Some of us swam daily in the local pool. We laughed and made it fun, pretending we were visiting a health club or spa rather than a hospital.

I continue to be motivated to pursue a daily exercise regime. I find that it helps in many ways, besides being a proven cancer preventative.

HEALING WATERS

When I was at home between chemo sessions, I continued the walks and the exercise regime. In the late afternoon and evening I often went swimming at Chico Hot Springs, a resort only five minutes from my home. I would soak in the hot pool and then swim a few laps in the larger, cooler pool. I would often listen to music or an inspirational or relaxing tape or read a book on healing. Sometimes I just pondered my own thoughts. At the beginning of the illness I did not feel like talking much to others, particularly if it involved explaining details about my illness. Later, I spent many happy hours chatting with friends while soaking in the warm, healing waters.

Sometimes I would visit Bozeman Hot Springs, about an hour's drive from home. This resort has a number of pools, from cold to very hot. I saw people going back and forth from one pool to another, and I started to do the same. I began a routine of dipping myself in the hot and cold pools seven times each. After the initial shock I came to enjoy that ritual. (You can do a simple form of this in your shower every day by alternating hot and cold water.)

The hot water was refreshing, particularly after the breast and lymph-node surgery. (I waited until the doctor okayed me to go into a hot tub. I also initially avoided extreme heat on the right arm to avoid lymphedema after the lymph-node surgery.)

Stress and concerns about cancer would seem to melt away as I soaked in the hot water. But apart from the general sense of relaxation and well-being, there is also evidence that this can directly help to strengthen the immune system and fight cancer. Soaking in hot water has been shown to increase the activity of natural killer cells—an important part of the immune system in dealing with cancer. Cancer cells also seem to be more vulnerable to heat than normal, healthy cells.[5]

YOGA

For several months while I was doing chemotherapy, I had walked past a yoga studio in Bozeman, Montana. Each time I passed I had an urge to go in, but somehow I never did. I did not really want to be in a large or even a small class at this time, unless it was with other women with cancer.

One day I decided just to peek in, and I took a flier from the counter. I saw that Nancy Ruby, the owner of the studio, gave private lessons, and I decided to schedule one. When I finally went to see her, I was about to go through my fourth chemotherapy session. It turned out to be one of the most helpful classes that I took.

There are many kinds of yoga, and they typically include postures, breathing exercises, and meditation. I explained to Nancy that I was most interested right then in getting through chemotherapy. She helped me understand what my body was telling me and adapted her program accordingly. We had one session based mostly on breathing exercises combined with visualization and simple postures for relaxation.

A new issue of *Yoga Journal* had just arrived and it contained an article about yoga as a supportive therapy in cancer treatment.[6] Nancy photocopied the article for me. I returned for another session, which we taped so I could use it during my chemotherapy.

Nancy boosted my confidence and helped me feel more relaxed. I felt that these simple techniques were one reason the last chemotherapy session was the easiest of the four. I also found that through her reflective listening I was able to hear my body telling me it was time to stop the chemotherapy after the fourth session.

Yoga is an excellent way to deal with stress and tension. It calms the body, mind and spirit. It elevates mood and energy level, eases pain, increases flexibility and boosts the immune system. I still include simple yoga poses in my daily routine.

Breathing Exercises

A large component of yoga involves conscious breathing techniques. Colleen and the hospital staff also stressed the benefits of breathing exercises, including deep breathing. I found just the act of breathing deeply and consciously could relax me during meditation or my spiritual practices or even while in the elevator on my way to the next blood test or sitting in a waiting room. It was simple and easy to do, and it didn't cost anything.

Why does deep breathing make you feel energized? On the most obvious level, it increases the flow of oxygen in the blood. In the East, however, there is an understanding that how we breathe can affect the flow of the life-force itself. This energy is known as *prana*, a Sanskrit term meaning "breath of life." The concept is similar to the Chinese understanding of *ch'i*, the energy that circulates through the body on the acupuncture meridians.

This universal energy force moves through the body with each breath, revivifying the organs and their related systems. Prana is absorbed most easily from the air, and exercise and deep breathing therefore increase the flow of prana through the body. Yoga, T'ai Chi and similar forms of exercise are specifically intended to increase the flow of this energy, which is most concentrated in the spiritual centers along the spine. These centers take in prana and distribute it through the body.

Those who practice healing methods of the East believe that sickness is the result of blocks or imbalances in the flow of this energy. Acupuncture and similar systems seek to remove blocks and balance this flow, with the understanding that when the proper flow of energy is restored, healing will occur.

I have found that deep breathing relaxes the body and brings about a healing state of calm, quietness and peace that can be tangibly felt. (And we have all experienced that a stuffy room is not conducive to good health.) The best source of health-giving prana is said to be "clean air near moving water, charged with sunlight."[7] I have certainly felt revitalized when standing near a fast-flowing waterfall not far from my home.

Another way of understanding this life-force is as the essence of the Holy Spirit that we take in through the breath. ("And the LORD God formed man of the dust of the ground, and breathed into his nostrils the breath of life; and man became a living soul."—Genesis 2:7)

CHECKLIST: WHY EXERCISE?

If you find it hard to get motivated to exercise, look at the following checklist. Regular moderate exercise for thirty minutes a day, or even every second day, has these beneficial effects:

- ✓ Boosts your immune system
- ✓ Helps normalize body weight
- ✓ Gets rid of excess fat, a known risk factor in many cancers
- ✓ Gets the blood and lymph fluid circulating
- ✓ Helps the body get rid of toxins
- ✓ Lifts your spirits
- ✓ Helps with depression and anxiety
- ✓ Helps you think
- ✓ Enhances your spirituality
- ✓ Increases vitality
- ✓ Helps control high blood pressure
- ✓ Reduces the risk of diabetes
- ✓ Reduces your risk of cancer by nearly 50%
- ✓ Helps you deal with the side effects of cancer treatment

CHAPTER 11

COMPLEMENTARY MEDICINE

From my research and experience, I could not find one single complementary or alternative treatment, or even a combination of treatments, that I felt could rightfully take the place of conventional treatment for my breast cancer. Having said that, complementary medicine was a powerful tool for me during my healing process. I found it particularly useful in dealing with the effects of chemotherapy and radiation and during my recovery from surgery.

From a spiritual perspective, just as I saw food as a means of delivering spiritual light to my body, I saw each herb or remedy or treatment as a means to provide my body with the healing light that it needed. When you look at it this way, the particular cup or "chalice" that the light comes in is not so important. It is all a matter of which delivery system works for you. Just as I might use a favorite mug for a herbal or green tea, I also might choose a fine teacup. What relieves the patient's thirst is really the contents of the vessel. We could debate all day about which cup is better, but it is the contents, the light, that performs the healing.

I believe, as do many patients, therapists, and more and more members of the medical profession, that complementary methods can be very helpful in the treatment of cancer. I know firsthand that these treatments can assist the body and the mind as well as the emotions. They also smoothed the rough edges of the traditional treatments for me.

I would not recommend complementary therapies as a replacement for proper medical care or accurate diagnosis, but these therapies can be wonderful adjuncts to healing. For example, a symptom of tiredness can mean a number of things in a cancer patient. It could be caused by the cancer itself, it could be a side effect of the treatment, or it could have a psychological component from the stress and anxiety of being diagnosed with a life-threatening disease. Conventional medicine has limited options to deal with these kinds of issues, but there are numerous complementary therapies that address low energy levels in the body.

NO MATTER WHAT YOUR ODDS ARE, COMPLEMENTARY THERAPIES SHOULD BE ABLE TO INCREASE YOUR SURVIVAL ODDS AND IMPROVE YOUR QUALITY OF LIFE.
—David Bognar

There are many different complementary techniques and products available, and you could end up spending a lot of time, energy, and money treating your body. My advice is to be selective. I turned down far more methods than I adopted.

That was sometimes hard to do, especially when a friend or relative lovingly offered something because of a desire to see me healed.

Sometimes I tried things that did not really appeal to me, particularly in those early days. I thought, "What have I got to lose?" or "Maybe they will help." But in the end, I did not continue with many of them. There is only so much that you can do and take each day and there is only so much that your body can absorb. Second, and probably more importantly, for something to work for me, I have to believe in it.

David Bognar, author of *Cancer: Increasing Your Odds for Survival*, outlines a useful approach to adding complementary therapies to conventional treatment for cancer. He says, "The first step in choosing an alternative treatment is knowing your odds with conventional treatment.... No matter what your odds are, complementary therapies should be able to increase your survival odds and improve your quality of life. As with any treatment, however, do not rush to action before you have done your homework."[1]

The book has a starter list of questions to ask yourself as you consider an alternative therapy or approach. The most useful for me were:

- Do you believe in the approach?
- Does it fit with your belief system?
- Do you have the time to do what is required?
- Can you afford it?[2]

Believing in a healing method really does make a difference. Bernie Siegel advises, "The most important thing is to pick a therapy you believe in and proceed with a positive attitude. Each person must chart his own course. One may want a comprehensive nutrition supplement program, while another thinks taking dozens of pills a day is too much of a nuisance, and it becomes counterproductive. Some can just 'leave their troubles to God' and be healed. Others need what I call the 'football coach' method, in which the patient plans every detail."[3]

THE MOST IMPORTANT THING IS TO PICK A THERAPY YOU
BELIEVE IN AND PROCEED WITH A POSITIVE ATTITUDE.
EACH PERSON MUST CHART HIS OWN COURSE.
—Dr. Bernie Siegel

After my research on alternatives, I chose those that seemed most appropriate for me. I prayed and asked for direction and often felt a sense of the rightness of each product or treatment that I used.

Some of the methods that assisted me most were Chinese and Western herbs, acupuncture, homeopathy, Bach Flower and other flower remedies, essential oils, chiropractic, and therapeutic massage. I will include here some notes on these so you can see why I made the choices I did. After doing your own research, choose what seems right for you and your individual program. You may apply the same principles and end up with a very different list. Every cancer is different, and every patient is different.

(These remedies can usually be used safely in conjunction with standard medical treatments. However, some remedies can interfere with the action of certain medications, so be sure to let your medical doctor *and* your naturopath know about *all* the medications you are taking—both traditional and complementary.)

HERBS

Douglas Schar, herbalist and author, has a balanced philosophy about herbs: "Preventive medicine is where herbal medicine makes its greatest contribution. There are no orthodox drugs available that prevent heart disease the way garlic or Hawthorne can. There are no synthesized pharmaceuticals that can prevent the common cold the way Echinacea or *maitake* can. These fascinating substances represent herbal medicine's unique contribution to the world of medicine and, indeed, to the future of medicine in general. If you have appendicitis, take yourself to the emergency room. If you want to avoid getting appendicitis, investigate herbal medicine."[4]

His comments echoed my thoughts about breast cancer. Now that I had the problem, I had no hesitation undergoing surgery to remove it. And yet, I was certainly interested in how herbs could help me deal with any side effects of treatment and prevent the condition returning.

There are a lot of herbs on the market, and you can spend a lot of time—and a lot of money—swallowing pills and drinking teas. Some say that what you mostly get is expensive urine. I am not so skeptical, having used herbs during my illness.

There are many useful books on herbs to get you started. One succinct and easy-to-read book is *Therapeutic Herb Manual: A Guide to the Safe and Effective Use of Liquid Herbal Extracts,* by Ed Smith, well-known medical herbalist and founder of Herb Pharm, an organic herb farm and herbal-extract company.

Herbalist Susan Weed's book *Breast Cancer? Breast Health!* has an interesting perspective on the use of herbs in breast cancer and describes how herbs can be used to support the body through all kinds of treatment, including radiation and chemotherapy. She stresses the importance of fresh herbs and cautions about herbs that have been sitting on a supermarket shelf for a long time. Health food stores or stores that specialize in selling herbs may be a better choice.

If you want to know all about herbs and cancer, read *Herbs Against Cancer: History and Controversy,* by Dr. Ralph Moss. This is a serious book about herbs from a historical and clinical perspective. He points out the fallacies and concerns about some of the popularly-touted herbs that are supposed to cure cancer.

I do believe that for some people these products may indeed work, and I do not doubt that some people have been cured by herbs and herbal remedies. In fact, my herbalist cured her husband of kidney cancer with the use of herbs. He completely trusted her with his care, and she delivered.

However, in the long run I felt I could not entrust my health to herbs alone. I researched everything that I could find, and if I had found one herb or combination that seemed to have a track record and work consistently, I certainly would have taken it. This would have been a lot more convenient than chemotherapy and radiation. However, my intuition told me that this was not going to be the case with me, and I think that this is true for most people. So instead of looking for herbs to "cure" my cancer, I used them as an adjunct to my treatment. I told the herbalist exactly what I was looking for—support for my immune system and assistance with the side effects of the medical treatment.

Not long after I began researching herbs, I met a herbalist at a store that sold herbs in bulk. She heard me ask about a specific hard-to-find herb that I had read about, and we started talking. After a consultation, she made up four specific herbal tinctures for me to use during the course of my illness. One was to boost my immune system, one to assist in digestion, one was a specific tincture for my constitution, and the fourth was to help with the effects of chemotherapy. These remedies included herbs that are not commonly found in over-the-counter medicines and capsules.

For example, the one for the immune system contained Baptisia, Phytolacca, Scrophularia, Turmeric, Thuja and Arctium. The digestive tincture contained Berberis, Xanthoxylum, Fouqueria, and Glycerrhiza. The tincture for chemotherapy contained Guta Kola, Ginkgo, Rosemary, Skullcap, Passion Flower, and Calamus. These herbs were very helpful for the "brain fog" of chemotherapy, a phenomenon that is well-known to cancer patients and the medical staff who care for them. Your brain feels kind of like cotton wool, and it is hard to concentrate, think, or focus, even on reading a book. I also used Ginkgo Biloba and Saint John's Wort to help keep my mind clear during chemotherapy.

I liked to know what the herbs were supposed to do so that I could visualize them doing their work. I took them in capsule form or in a tea, tincture, or herbal extract. Some other herbs I used during chemotherapy and radiation included Astragalus, Yellow Dock, Siberian Ginseng, Milk Thistle, and Burdock root, which are known to boost the immune system and to boost white and red blood cells. Milk Thistle improves liver function and protects the liver, which is the main organ that metabolizes and removes chemotherapy agents from the system. I also used a Chinese herbal remedy called Curing Pills (a traditional formula containing sixteen different Chinese herbs) to help with nausea and gastrointestinal upsets during chemotherapy. Another supplement that helps normalize the functioning of the digestive system after chemotherapy is acidophilus, which restores the body's natural intestinal flora.

Another helpful herbal product I found was Saint John's Wort oil, which I used on my skin to reduce the inflammation sometimes caused by radiation therapy. I applied it overnight to the breasts and washed it off in the morning, before the next treatment. I found it to be very effective.

Some herbs can interfere with the action of certain medications, so be sure to let your doctor know which herbs you are taking.

MELATONIN
Melatonin, a hormone that is secreted by the pineal gland, is involved in regulating sleep and the daily rhythm of the body's functions. As a supplement, it is gaining popularity in breast-cancer treatment for its ability to enhance the immune system.

Although it is available over the counter in health food stores and drug stores, you should consult your doctor before self-treating, as it does have side effects and can interact with some drugs. It can also cause problems with certain illnesses and is not appropriate for women who are pregnant, breastfeeding, or considering pregnancy. Its long-term safety is unknown. I took it for over a year during my treatment and continue to take it daily as an antioxidant.[5]

GREEN TEA EXTRACT

For thousands of years Eastern medicine has extolled the benefits of green tea, and today it is known for its ability to promote general health and well being. Green tea extract protects against oxidative stress caused by free radicals, promotes healthy cholesterol levels and supports the immune system. The naturopaths at CTCA recommend either nine cups of green tea per day or green tea capsules (an easier way to get your antioxidant boost).

TURMERIC OR CURCUMIN

Curcumin is the active ingredient in the Indian spice turmeric, often used in curry. Research suggests that curcumin has powerful antioxidant properties and promotes healthy cellular division. It is known for strengthening the immune system and research suggests that it supports liver detoxification, thus speeding excretion of toxic compounds. Laboratory experiments at MD Anderson Cancer Center showed it to be a powerful agent against cancer cells.[6] The naturopaths at CTCA now incorporate this into their treatment regimen for breast cancer patients. I took it during my treatment and have added a capsule a day to my cancer prevention regimen.

MODIFIED CITRUS PECTIN

Modified Citrus Pectin (MCP), also known as fractionated pectin, is produced from the peel or pulp of oranges, grapefruits, and lemons, and it is usually taken in powder form mixed with water or juice. It has demonstrated unique properties in preventing the spread of cancer through metastasis.[7]

At a cellular level, Modified Citrus Pectin acts to block cancer cell aggregation, adhesion, and metastasis. It attaches to cancer cells to prevent them from spreading throughout the body. It is said to promote healthy immune system functioning and helps to maintain the growth of normal cells, while supporting healthy tissue.

I took Modified Citrus Pectin during my second bout of breast cancer at the recommendation of the naturopaths at the Cancer Treatment Centers of America. It is a safe and inexpensive way to reduce the risk of metastasis—and in many types of cancer, distant metastases are much more life-threatening than the primary tumor.

HOMEOPATHY

In the 1980s, I attended a seminar by medical doctor and well-respected homeopath Bill Gray. From the beginning, I appreciated the holistic approach of homeopathy and its subtle yet profound effects on body, mind, and emotions—and even on the soul.

When you first hear about it, homeopathy can seem puzzling. The word *homeopathy* is derived from the Greek words meaning "similar" and "suffering." It literally means "treatment by similars." It is based on the "law of similars," which states that a substance that causes certain symptoms in a healthy person can cure the same symptoms in an unhealthy one.

For example, if a substance has been found to cause nausea in a healthy person, when you give that same substance in minute quantities to a person suffering from nausea, it alleviates their symptoms. (There are correspondences to the law of similars in traditional medicine: allergies are treated with a tiny dose of allergen, and immunizations are given using a tiny dose of a pathogen.)

That homeopathic remedies are given in tiny doses seems to go against the grain in our society, where more is better. However, homeopathy has been around for over two hundred years and has been documented to show significant benefits. It rarely causes side effects and is often less expensive than pharmaceuticals.

Although no one really knows how homeopathy works, many people think it has a spiritual component. Like Chinese medicine and other complementary therapies, it includes the concepts that illness is the result of imbalances in the life-force within the body. The remedies do not try to suppress symptoms but rather influence the subtle balance of energy in the whole body. A homeopathic remedy tries to go to the cause of a condition by stimulating the healing energies within the body itself. An experienced homeopath sees you and your body as unique. Homeopathic practitioners take a detailed history and perform a comprehensive assessment of your mental and emotional state as well as your physical symptoms. They will recommend one or more remedies based on this complete picture of your consitition and current mental, emotional and physical state. (This is a more holistic approach than the conventional scientific one, which often seeks to isolate specific components of an illness and treat them individually.)

Because they work with the finer energies in the body, many of the most successful homeopaths are quite intuitive. I have noticed that good diagnosticians in any field—whether traditional or alternative health practitioners or even a car mechanic—often have a sixth sense about a problem that guides them to the right solution, even when the outer evidence may be inconclusive.

This intuition is something we all posses in varying degrees, and even if we are not an expert in a particular field, our intuition can certainly help guide us to find the right practitioners. Beyond recognizing their excellent knowledge and superior skills, we often have a "good feeling" about them, there is something that inspires trust. I think we need to learn to take notice of our good and bad feelings about those whom we trust with our care. I believe that our Higher Self often guides us through those feelings. When I have ignored them in the past, I have regretted it.

Another approach to homeopathy is a more do-it-yourself method. Instead of going to an experienced practitioner for a constitutional remedy, many people self-medicate for minor complaints and symptoms. For example, I often use an over-the-counter homeopathic cold remedy. I used Arnica Montana in the form of a homeopathic cream on the site of any punctures made for blood tests and intravenous lines to prevent bruising and assist in healing. I also used Carbo Vegetabilis and Arsenicum Album to help deal with nausea during chemotherapy. (However, the naturopaths that I spoke to said that the nausea of chemotherapy is very intense and not easily treated by homeopathy.)

This symptomatic use of homeopathic remedies can be very helpful. However, for the best results with more challenging issues and to go to a deeper level of healing, this is not a substitute for seeing someone who is an expert and can tailor the remedies to your unique situation.[*]

I do not see homeopathy as a replacement for traditional medical care for a serious condition. I used homeopathic remedies to deal with more subtle energetic issues underlying the condition, to help in my overall wellness program and to counter side effects of treatment.

BACH FLOWER REMEDIES

In the 1930s, Dr. Edward Bach, a physician, bacteriologist, and pathologist, developed a system to heal the emotional imbalance behind disease using water specially prepared with different English wildflowers. Bach's remedies are used to help with emotional well-being, mind-body health, and even the development of the soul.

"Heal thyself" is at the heart of Dr. Bach's philosophy. He said, "Disease is solely and purely corrective; it is neither vindictive nor cruel, but it is the means adopted by our own souls to point out to us our faults, to prevent our making greater errors, to hinder us from doing more harm, and to bring us back to the path of Truth and Light from which we never should have strayed."[8] I have appreciated Bach Flower Remedies for some years for their ability to help me find balance in body, mind, and spirit.

One of Dr. Bach's most well-known formulas is Rescue Remedy, composed of five different flower essences. It is used for stressful situations or medical emergencies such as accident, sudden bad news, bereavement, or situations where a patient is going into shock. It can even be used before a difficult meeting or before taking a test—any situation that can raise your stress level. Like all Bach Flower Remedies,

---

[*] One homeopath has told me that patients who have had cancer should not take the homeopathic remedy Silica, as it could potentially release residual cancer cells from old scar tissue and cause a recurrence.

Rescue Remedy is not intended to replace medical treatment, but it can provide invaluable support while waiting for medical help in an emergency. It is natural, safe, and gentle and will not interfere with any form of medical treatment. Even prior to my diagnosis, I carried Rescue remedy in my purse or briefcase for use in emergencies.

Flower essences are similar to homeopathic remedies in that they do not work because of the chemical composition of the remedy. Flower essences are *vibrational* in nature and they work through the energy field that is imparted to the substance of the remedy in its preparation. Bach developed thirty-eight different remedies, each one designed to bring a particular mental or emotional state back into balance. Ann Louise Gittleman calls them "psychotherapy in a bottle."[9] I believe that they work on the finer bodies with the help of the Higher Self.

As I used these remedies, I found that they had subtle but profound effects on my mood, emotions, thought processes, and personal psychology. I would not notice anything initially, but perhaps a few hours or days later I would notice that my outlook on life had changed.

I bought a few of the many books that describe the flower remedies and the specific action of each one. I prayed and asked to be shown the right remedy. Often when I opened the book, the first one I saw would seem to match exactly what I needed at that time. Here are some that helped me in my healing journey.[10]

Olive

Dr. Bach described Olive as the remedy for "those who have suffered much mentally or physically and are so exhausted and weary that they feel they have no more strength to make any effort. Daily life is hard for them, without pleasure."[11] The remedy helps to restore enthusiasm for life. It helps you tap into a higher source and thereby find new energy and restoration at all levels.

Elm

Elm is for those who "suddenly feel overwhelmed by their responsibilities and feel inadequate to deal with them or keep up with events; this is often brought about by taking on too much work without taking care of oneself. As a result they feel depressed and exhausted, with a temporary loss of self-esteem."[12] The remedy helps you find balance in your life, setting realistic expectations and goals. It also helps you to be open to receiving assistance from others and from the Higher Self, instead of relying exclusively on the energies of the ego and the lower self. When you are "overwhelmed by responsibility," as many cancer patients feel, this remedy can help find a new perspective and determine a practical course of action.

Walnut

Walnut is a remedy specifically to help in dealing with change of any sort: divorce, marriage, change in career, menopause, or any change in circumstances. I often use Walnut for dealing with jet lag and the general effects of long-distance travel. Anyone who has been diagnosed with cancer is already facing a major change, and many people facing this situation find that they want to make changes in a number of areas of their life as part of their healing. Walnut can help you navigate through change in a positive way, following your inner direction, while at the same time protecting you from negative external influences.

I bought my own kit of the Bach Flower Remedies and made my own little bottles of remedies from the stock bottles. I would tailor my own formula from several different remedies that met my needs at that time. Every week or so, I would see how I was doing and change the formula if I had made progress in some areas or if new issues had arisen.

One combination that I used to alleviate feelings of discouragement, despondency, and fear included Mimulus, Cherry Plum, Aspen, Agrimony, Gentian, and Mustard. Mimulus is known for helping you face difficulties with courage and confidence; Cherry Plum helps you think calmly and rationally; Aspen helps to replace fear and worry with confidence; Agrimony helps you communicate your feelings and see problems in perspective; and Gentian and Mustard bring hope when there is discouragement and despair.

FLOWER ESSENCES

Dr. Bach's original remedies using English wildflowers are the most popular and widely-known flower essences, but other people have developed other flower-essence remedies based on the same principles. I have tried some of the new formulas based on North American wildflowers and found them to be very helpful. I took Yarrow and Pink Yarrow to help set appropriate boundaries in my life and promote the healing of the inner child, or the soul.

Yarrow

Yarrow helps those who are easily depleted or tend to absorb negative influences from their environment. The description of Yarrow in *Flower Essence Repertory,* by Patricia Kaminski and Richard Katz, explains how this essence may work from a spiritual standpoint.

"Those who typically need this remedy are easily affected by their surroundings and can be prone to many forms of environmental illness, allergies, or psychosomatic diseases. Such persons have an extraordinary capacity for healing, counseling, or teaching, because they are readily able to receive the psychic information and to understand the pain and suffering of others. At the same time, they are easily depleted and are quite vulnerable to the thoughts or negative intentions of others. Yarrow literally 'knits together' the overly porous aura of such an individual so that the aura does not 'bleed' so excessively into its environment. Furthermore, it helps such a person re-balance and stabilize the abundant light which radiates in the upper energy centers, directing it into the lower centers so that the Self has more vitality and solidity.... Yarrow bestows a shining shield of light which protects and unifies the essential Self, allowing compassionate healing qualities to flow freely from one's soul to others."[13]

This description resonated for me and for other cancer patients whom I knew when I shared it with them. Breast-cancer patients in particular are known for their caring and often overly self-giving nature.

I used this remedy successfully to help me concentrate on my own healing and not get too tied up in other patients and their illnesses. This is a common concern for doctors, counselors, teachers, healers, and ministers, who may have a great capacity for healing but tend to become depleted of energy and take on the pain and suffering of others.

The beneficial effects of this essence and of my own internal work during my cancer treatment have been lasting, and I find that I now have a greater capacity to set loving boundaries and not give of myself until I am depleted, which often happened to me as a doctor and as a minister.

Pink Yarrow

The properties of Pink Yarrow are similar to those of Yarrow. It is especially known for helping the individual distinguish between true compassion and overly sympathetic identification with others.

I found Yarrow and Pink Yarrow useful when I entered the hospital environment, which can be very draining to many patients. Although hospitals are dedicated to healing, they often lack a truly healing environment for those who are in them—they are busy places, full of sick and worried people.

Yarrow Special Formula

I also used a remedy called Yarrow Special Formula. This remedy contains flower essences of Yarrow, Arnica, and Echinacea with fresh tinctures of these plants in a base of seawater. It was originally developed in 1986 after the Chernobyl accident to help heal the body and strengthen the aura when dealing with the harmful effects of nuclear radiation.[14] I used this formula while undergoing radiation therapy to help minimize negative effects from exposure to the radiation.

ESSENTIAL OILS

Essential oils are mentioned in the Bible and many of the sacred scriptures of the world's religions. They are distilled from the roots, leaves, flowers, and other parts of plants. They have been used for centuries in perfumes and to promote health and well-being. Essential oils have many restorative effects on the body. They are used to relax muscles, stimulate circulation, relieve pain, enhance immunity, alleviate physical, mental, and emotional stress, and fight infection. They can support the body, mind, and spirit and help strengthen the body so that it can heal itself.

I can feel the effect of an essential oil within a few seconds of applying it to my body or even just smelling it. Essential oils have a wonderfully uplifting and subtle effect on the body as well as the spirit, the mind, and the emotions. I used them to assist the healing process and to smooth out the effects of surgery or treatment.

The plants used to produce high-quality essential oils are grown organically and carefully harvested. These oils are expensive because they are pure and don't contain synthetic compounds or fillers. However, the pure, natural oils are more effective healing agents, so it is worth spending the extra money for them. Fortunately, the pure oils are highly concentrated and are used sparingly, so they last a long time. They are usually diluted before use by placing five or six drops into an ounce of unscented lotion or carrier oil, such as almond oil.

Oils can be applied during massage, through compresses, or directly to the body. They can be used in baths or inhaled after being diffused into the air. They can be applied to the pulse points or to any specific area of the body that needs attention. I often placed them on my heart or over the third eye, the spiritual center in the brow. An easy way to use them is to place a drop in your hand and rub your palms together, smelling the fragrance as you do.

When essential oils are diffused into the air, the compounds in the oil stimulate the olfactory nerve, which is connected to areas deep within the brain. This can directly influence mood, emotions, and many of the unconscious functions of the body. When used in a bath or for massage, they are directly absorbed through the skin and can affect every part of the body within twenty minutes. Here are some of the oils that I used during my cancer treatment. I still use these and other oils today.[15]

Neroli

Since I was a child, I have known that my name, Neroli, is the name of an essential oil derived from the orange blossom. It is named after a princess from the town of Nerola, Italy, who used the oil and began the practice of using orange blossoms in bridal bouquets.

As I began to study essential oils, I found out about the healing properties of this oil. It is used to lift depression and anxiety, to calm and relax the body (including the muscles), and to deal with stress. It has powerful effects on the psychology. It helps to bring things into focus and helps us to be present in the moment. It can be used to strengthen and stabilize the emotions and bring relief to seemingly hopeless situations.

As I read about the uses of this oil, I realized that its healing properties matched my needs perfectly. I really got the message when two different friends sent me neroli oil in the same week.

Frankincense

Frankincense is an ancient oil. It has long been known for its antiseptic properties, and it is also used today for its ability to stimulate the immune system. It is a calming and holy oil—frankincense was one of the gifts given to Christ at his birth. I was familiar with frankincense as an incense and for its use in improving communication with the Creator, but I did not know of its anti-tumor properties until a fellow minister pointed them out to me.

Frankincense has been found to increase the activity of white blood cells and is thought to improve the immune system through several different means. It is also said to promote spiritual awareness, assist with meditation, and give you the kind of attitude adjustment that is very helpful when facing a challenging illness or disease.

Lavender

Lavender is used to balance the body. It is said to promote a sense of well-being and has been used traditionally to treat many different conditions. It is often used to decrease inflammation and infection and to lift depression. It has soothing and regenerating properties and is wonderfully relaxing in baths and in massage.

Spikenard

Spikenard oil is a personal favorite. It is used in India as a medicinal herb and to nourish and regenerate the skin. But this oil is also known for its spiritual properties and its ability to assist the soul through difficult initiations. It is recorded in the Bible that Mary Magdalene used this holy oil to anoint Jesus before the Last Supper, and Jesus explained that this was in preparation for his burial—for his passing through the initiations of the crucifixion and the resurrection. It is used to help the soul pass through the dark night of the soul and the dark night of the Spirit. I have come to love its distinctive fragrance.

Peppermint

Peppermint has long been known to sooth the digestive system. It is used to help reduce nausea during chemotherapy. It has also been reputed to improve concentration and mental acuity.

Other Essential Oils

During my treatment I also used a number of blends of oils produced by Young Living, a company that specializes in high-quality essential oils.

White Angelica and Gathering helped at difficult times when I felt I needed strengthening in order to deal with chaotic or negative energies—and when the chemotherapy agents were going in, it could indeed feel like a bombardment of negative energy. Gathering also helped me to focus my energies, and I often used it before consultations with the oncologist and at other times when I needed to be fully attentive.

Harmony is a blend including neroli, rose, and sandalwood oils. I found that it was soothing and helped to reduce stress and create an overall sense of well-being.

CHIROPRACTIC

Although we do not fully understand the biochemistry of touch, we do know that human beings need it and respond to it. Chiropractic and massage are two ways that touch can heal the body.

There are many kinds of chiropractic treatment, but in general, chiropractic treats the musculoskeletal system in order to bring balance and alignment to the body and the nervous system. According to current theories , subtle changes in the motion of the vertebrae can have a profound impact on the complex system of nerves that run through and alongside the vertebrae.

Chiropractic can stimulate the production of endorphins, the body's natural pain relievers, and can free blocked energy within the body in a way similar to acupuncture. Many chiropractors combine spinal manipulation with other alternative disciplines, such as nutrition, relaxation therapies, and Chinese herbal medicine.

If I ever have back pain, or if my back feels like it is "out," the chiropractor is the first person I want to see. But even if I don't have an immediate problem, I like to see a chiropractor on a regular basis to assist in keeping my body "tuned" and in balance.

MASSAGE

There are many different types of massage. Therapeutic massage helps eliminate toxins, align bones, muscles and ligaments, and restore motion in joints. It can help improve the circulation of blood and lymph fluid in the body, which can help the immune system. It can also stimulate the nervous system and alleviate stress. Massage is intended to boost the intrinsic healing ability of the body. At key times in my cancer treatment, I found that massage helped to reduce stress levels and promote healing. Some forms of massage also aim at freeing energy blocks at deeper levels of the body, stimulating change on emotional and other levels of being. Although I did not look for this, it sometimes happened and was helpful.

Patients with cancer need to be careful about massage, especially deep-tissue massage. Check first with your doctor. This is particularly true for breast cancer patients who have had surgery to the lymph system. Professionally trained therapists will always check your medical history and adjust their treatment accordingly.

ACUPUNCTURE

The ancient Chinese practice of acupuncture uses fine needles inserted at specific points on the meridians of the body. According to the theories of acupuncture, the meridians are pathways through which vital energy, known as *ch'i*, flows to the organs and the whole body.

While acupuncture meridians do not correspond to any known physical system of the body, they do mirror, energetically or spiritually, the flow of blood in the circulatory system and electrical impulses in the nervous system. In fact, a diagram of the meridians in the body looks very similar to a chart of the vascular or nervous systems, even to the untrained eye. If there is abundant and unobstructed flow of energy through the meridians, then we have a healthy body and increased vitality. The aim of the treatments is to remove blocks and normalize the flow of energy on the meridians.

I had several sessions of acupuncture, and like many patients, I would often feel a sense of well-being and relaxation during and after a treatment. It was an interesting feeling of being relaxed and energized at the same time. The treatment also brought a pleasant feeling of warmth to the area being treated, a sign of increased flow of circulation and energy to that area. Insertion of the needles usually causes very little pain, since they are very fine. Like many holistic treatments, acupuncture also seems to affect the mind and emotions as well as the physical body.

Scientific studies have confirmed that acupuncture can be very effective in helping to control nausea resulting from chemotherapy.[16] Although I did not use it for this purpose as it was not available at the hospital at that time, one patient I knew relied heavily on acupuncture during her chemotherapy. She would leave the doctor's office after her injection and go straight to her acupuncturist. She swears that she had a much easier time with chemotherapy because of his treatments; she certainly noticed the difference if she missed a session.

Many cancer treatment centers now offer acupuncture as part of their complementary medicine programs. I used it while receiving treatment for my recurrence and found its ability to alleviate physical symptoms to be remarkable.

Acupuncture, like most forms of medicine, is an art as well as a science, so it pays to seek out a skilled and intuitive practitioner. Certification requirements for acupuncturists vary widely in different jurisdictions, so look for one who is certified by a recognized national body, such as the National Certification Commission for Acupuncture and Oriental Medicine. And of course, make sure that they use only disposable needles.

Choosing a Practitioner

I believe that the healing power of massage and other hands-on treatment methods comes in part from the person delivering the treatment, in part from the Higher Self of the practitioner, and in part from the Higher Self of the one being treated. There is a flow of energy during the healing process that is a science as well as an art, and it obeys natural laws, just like the laws of physics.

There are definitely therapists who have "healing hands." Therapists who are connected and centered with their Higher Self can transmit a healing current through their hands during a treatment. On the other hand, if a therapist is depressed or unhappy or angry, this negative energy can also be passed on to the patient; even worse, the therapist can drain positive energy from the patient.

Doctors, therapists, healers, and health workers can also take on negative energy from patients (whether consciously or subconsciously) if they do not know how to seal their own auric forcefield. This is one reason why therapists wash their hands between patients. Apart from being good hygiene, it also helps to remove any negative energies that the therapist may have picked up. The water breaks the contact and is a means of clearing the aura as well as cleaning the physical body.

I also know from experience how easy it is to feel drained after seeing many different patients. One way this can occur is if the therapist transfers to a patient some of the finite energy of their own auric forcefield, instead of simply being the conduit for the energies of the Higher Self, which are not limited.

In general, I am selective when it comes to letting people touch my body for treatment. If a therapist is tired or out of sorts, I may decide to forgo treatment that day—energy may flow from me to them, and that it not the purpose of the treatment. If I do not like the look or the vibration of the person, if they are angry or inharmonious, then I do not want that energy to be transferred to my body, and I may look for someone else. I always ask the angels to lead me to the right person—and they seem to do so.

I pray before practitioners place their hands on me that only the light of their Higher Self will pass to me and that none of the energies of my lesser self will pass to them. I also ask the angels, including my guardian angel, to work with them to align my body and to perform any adjustment necessary.

OTHER THERAPIES

I have mentioned here some of the complementary therapies that worked for me in my cancer treatment. There are other complementary therapies I have used in the past and that I have found effective (for example, reflexology and Ayurvedic medicine) which I did not choose to use for this particular illness. I could not do everything, so I simply chose the methods that felt right for me at that time. You or a loved one may choose other therapies that you feel will work for you.

There are a multitude of different complementary therapies available. Be selective—you cannot try them all. Take your time—for you do have time to do your homework. Get help if you need it, but ultimately the choice is yours. There are a number of comprehensive and well-researched books that outline the many different options. I looked for ones that had solid scientific data to show what really works. Do your research and follow your heart.

CHECKLIST: CHOOSING COMPLEMENTARY THERAPIES

✓ **Combine complementary therapies with traditional medicine.**

✓ **Choose alternative health practitioners that you feel good about.**

✓ **Consider therapies for each of these areas:**

    ○ Fight the cancer

    ○ Support your immune system

    ○ Cope with the effects of treatment

✓ **Be selective.** You can't do everything.

✓ **Do your research.** Is there solid evidence and studies to show that a particular therapy is effective and increases your odds for survival?

✓ **Ask yourself:**

    ○ Do I believe in the approach?

    ○ Does it fit with my belief system?

    ○ Do I have the time to do what is required?

    ○ Can I afford it?

✓ **Remember, ultimately it is your choice.**

    ○ Ask for guidance.

    ○ Follow your heart.

CHAPTER 12

LIFESTYLE AND ENVIRONMENTAL CHANGES

The final part of my physical program for healing included environmental and lifestyle changes. It is well known these days that pollutants in food, water, and the environment are one cause of cancer. But even apart from their direct carcinogenic effects, these substances place an added burden on the immune system. The immune system has to identify them, and the liver, kidneys, and other organs have to process them and remove them from the body.

Modern science tends to try to isolate individual factors when looking for the causes of cancer, and this approach does have value. However, specialists in environmental medicine speak about the "total load" on the immune system as a key cause of concern. There may be no single pollutant that is harmful or fatal by itself, but each puts a certain load on the immune system, and the total may be more than the body can effectively handle.

Either way, it made sense to do what I could to remove unnecessary toxins and chemicals from my environment. Just having the tumor removed in the lumpectomy was one less thing that my immune system had to deal with. Anything else I could do to unburden my immune system would free it up for the challenges of chemotherapy and radiation and dealing with any residual cancer cells that might cause a recurrence.

I consider myself very fortunate to live in a mountain environment with clean air and water, and thus I do not have to deal with many of the everyday pollution concerns that people in large cities face. Also, I did not smoke or drink alcohol (both of which put a burden on the immune system and have been shown to increase the risk of cancer). I now began to consider other environmental burdens that I might not have been aware of previously.

For example, I look for organically-grown foods, which are now becoming widely available in regular supermarkets. I now use only natural deodorants and try to use more natural cosmetics and personal-care products where there are good alternatives available. (I feel that avoiding artificial chemicals may be especially important in deodorants, which are applied to the skin very near the breast and directly over the lymph nodes that are nearest to the breast.)

WHEN LOOKING AT LIFESTYLE AND ENVIRONMENT, THINK
ABOUT THE TOTAL LOAD ON THE IMMUNE SYSTEM AND
HOW TO REDUCE IT.

There is also evidence that wearing a bra (especially an underwired bra) for more than twelve hours a day may increase the risk of breast cancer,[1] so I now try to make sure I have bras that are comfortable and fit well and don't cause irritation or unnecessarily restrict the flow of blood and lymph fluid.

I do not believe that any one of these factors causes breast cancer in itself, but if I can reduce the overall risk by a small percentage, I feel it is worthwhile, especially since having had one occurrence I have a statistically increased risk of future breast cancer.

With more and more natural and organic products available, it is not difficult to make these kinds of changes. Once again, it is not "all or nothing"—you don't have to go 100 percent organic to make a difference. Remember, it is the total load on the immune system that is the key, and any substitutions you make will help.

CHAPTER 13

MEDICINE AND THE MIND

The mind, body, and emotions are connected and they all affect the immune system. This connection is now being documented scientifically. Mind-body medicine techniques are being incorporated into many treatment programs for cancer and other illnesses in major medical centers, and many patients are seeking out these forms of therapy.

Dr. Joan Borysenko, author of *Minding the Body, Mending the Mind* and a leading researcher on the mind-body connection in medicine, says, "We've always known that we can literally die of broken hearts and shattered dreams. Laboratory findings are now corroborating that intuitive sense. The most pressing question for us, then, is how to reconnect with hope, faith, and love, and how to use these states for minding the body and mending the mind."[1]

I had been aware of the mind-body connection long before my own experience with cancer, as I had seen it at work in my patients years before. I remember one patient who was taking a number of different medications for hypertension and still having difficulty getting her blood pressure under control. She was even attending a specialist clinic at a university medical school, since her blood pressure would sometimes become dangerously high. One day she confided in me that the main source of stress in her life was her mother-in-law. I happened to be measuring her blood pressure at the time, and I saw it suddenly shoot up. We had discovered the real problem.

She described how she was very happily married, but her mother-in-law disliked her and tried to interfere in her life at every turn. Whenever she spoke or thought about this relative I would see her blood pressure go up twenty points. We experimented with this, and when she consciously calmed her emotions, her blood pressure would return to normal.

She was immediately motivated. When she worked on the relationship with her mother-in-law, or rather, in setting appropriate boundaries and not reacting to her mother-in-law, she was able to gradually reduce her medication under her specialist's direction. She could not change or control her mother-in-law, but with her husband's help, she could limit her influence in their lives. She could also change the way that she reacted to her mother-in-law. As well as dealing with the medical problem, she had learned a soul lesson that enabled her to live a happier and fuller life.

I found this kind of medicine very satisfying, since it could help people get to the real cause of their problems rather than just treat symptoms. I enjoyed spending more time with my patients, helping them to find out how they could help themselves. This was one reason why I was often behind with my schedule, and also one reason why my patients often did not mind waiting—they knew I would take the extra time with them, too, if it was needed.

I was also aware of the mind-body connection in my personal life. I believe that your attitude, thoughts, and feelings can make you well or can make you ill. Also, if you listen to your body, it will often tell you what it needs. I think that a part of the reason I was now facing cancer was that I had been ignoring the messages my body had been sending to me for some time. I knew that I had a problem when I observed how I first reacted to the diagnosis of cancer—a sense of relief that I did not have to return to work. I had also been sending my body some very negative messages for some time (for example, "This job is killing me") and my body had evidently followed this script obediently.

WE'VE ALWAYS KNOWN THAT WE CAN LITERALLY DIE OF BROKEN HEARTS AND SHATTERED DREAMS.... THE MOST PRESSING QUESTION FOR US, THEN, IS HOW TO RECONNECT WITH HOPE, FAITH, AND LOVE, AND HOW TO USE THESE STATES FOR MINDING THE BODY AND MENDING THE MIND.
—Dr. Joan Borysenko

Bernie Siegel says, "I personally feel that we do have biological 'live' and 'die' mechanisms within us. Other doctors' scientific research and my own day-to-day clinical experience have convinced me that the state of mind changes the state of the body by working through the central nervous system, the endocrine system, and the immune system. Peace of mind sends the body a 'live' message, while depression, fear, and unresolved conflict give it a 'die' message. Thus, all healing is scientific, even if science can't yet explain exactly how unexpected 'miracles' occur."[2]

As I faced my diagnosis, I realized that my body and mind now needed to follow a new set of directions—to live! I lost no time in sending this new message. I had a serious talk with my body, my body elemental, and my Higher Self. I let them all know that I had given some wrong directions that needed to be deleted. I asked them to replace these incorrect instructions with correct thoughtforms and healthy thoughts and feelings. And I said that I would be working closely with them from now on and would be providing the needed resources.

I realized I needed to get up to speed very quickly, so I turned to the study of mind-body medicine and psychoneuroimmunology (PNI)—a big word for a simple concept. It has three parts. *Psycho* refers to the mind—thought and emotional processes and mood states. *Neuro* refers to the neurological and neuroendocrine systems—the nervous system and the hormones. *Immunology* refers to the immune system and cellular functions.

Put it all together and PNI is a powerful means of using the mind and emotions working through the neurological systems to assist your immune system. There is much we still do not know about exactly how the mind-body connection works, but the connection is undeniable, and many patients and their families understand it instinctively.

ALL HEALING IS SCIENTIFIC, EVEN IF SCIENCE CAN'T YET
EXPLAIN EXACTLY HOW UNEXPECTED "MIRACLES" OCCUR.
—Dr. Bernie Siegel

IMAGERY FOR HEALING

There are many different ways in which the mind-body connection can be activated. One that I had known about for some time is the use of imagery in healing. I had read the work of Jeanne Achterberg, author of *Imagery in Healing,* and of Martin Rossman, author of *Health Through Imagery,* and had attended one of Dr. Rossman's lectures. I loved the stories of the visualizations that other patients used to boost their immune system and found, as I suspected, that the use of visualization in healing is very individual.

One popular way to use imagery in cancer treatment is to visualize the cancer cells in the body being dealt with on a cellular level. Some patients visualize all kinds of things eating up cancer cells—anything from sharks to vicious dogs to Pac-Man icons. Children often like to imagine a video game where they are blasting cancer cells with lasers or rockets. Those with a scientific background might visualize the action of the immune system and the white cells attacking and removing the cancer cells.

At first it seems unlikely that visualizing sharks eating cancer cells could make a difference. But somehow it seems that these activities of the mind do translate into a change in the activity of the body on a cellular level. We may not understand all the cause-and-effect sequences in this process, but the results are there.[3]

As I experimented with these techniques, I used my medical training to help me visualize healthy immune cells working and to see the cancer dissolving. I also used medical textbooks to visualize the anatomy of the area involved. Eventually, however, over the course of my treatment, my visualizations evolved and I found that I was most comfortable with imagery of a spiritual nature.

One of these visualizations was of violet light saturating the body. Violet is the color of change and transmutation, and I visualized this light dissolving the cancer and clearing the body of any burdens or negativity from any source. I also visualized the violet light working on my finer bodies—changing my thoughts and emotions to be more life-affirming and even changing the way I thought about cancer.

Another visualization used an emerald-green light—the healing green of nature that is healing to the eye, the soul, and the body. I visualized this light strengthening my healthy cells and my immune system, realigning all the cells and organs of the body into a state of perfect health.

The third visualization I used was a thoughtform of green, blue, and white light that is known as the healing thoughtform. This thoughtform is composed of concentric spheres—a sphere of white surrounded by a sphere of blue suspended within a globe of green. The white sphere represents purity and the dissolving of any negativity of the injured or ill part. The blue represents the original "blueprint" or perfect pattern of that organ or body part and how it is intended to function. The green sphere is the light of healing, which returns the cells and the organs to a state of wholeness.[4]

I spent some time each day visualizing the healing thoughtform over my breasts and heart and over my entire body, and I also included this thoughtform as part of my prayers. I prayed for this healing thoughtform to be placed over my physical, mental, emotional, and spiritual bodies as I visualized it doing its perfect work.

I simply prayed as follows: "In the name of my Higher Self, in the name of Mother Mary and Archangel Raphael, I ask for the healing thoughtform to be lowered over me and to heal all vestiges of breast cancer in my body. May it produce perfect healing of my body, mind, and soul. According to God's holy will, let it be done."

I had three pieces of fluorite crystal that I used to help me with my visualization. One was violet, one was green, and the third was carved in the shape of a heart with white, green, and violet all swirled together. I took them with me to chemotherapy treatments and would hold them as touchstones, physical reminders of my visualizations.

There are some very good books on the use of imagery in healing and the powerful effects it can have on the body. I have listed some of them in the resources at the end of the book. I found it liberating and empowering just to read them and to find out how much we can do, just with our thoughts and feelings, to bring about healing.

CANCER AND PSYCHOLOGY

Psychological therapy was a great support to my healing journey. So many emotions arise in cancer patients—not just the obvious ones of fear and depression but also guilt, anger, and resentment. If these emotions can be dealt with and positive emotions engaged, it can make a tremendous difference in how the body responds to the challenge of disease.

Norman Shealy, renowned neurosurgeon and founder of the American Holistic Medicine Association, says in his book *Sacred Healing*, "The bottom line is, *you cannot afford the luxury of fear, anxiety, anger, guilt, or depression,* no matter what the cause! And you can't afford prejudice, dislike, hatred, resentment, greed, or ignorance. At some level there has to be a physiological negative effect."[5]

It is well known that high blood pressure, heart attacks, and migraines are associated with chronic anger. Dr. Shealy points out something that is not so well known, however, which is that chronic depression is clearly associated medically with cancer.[6] (This does not mean that chronic depression causes cancer; rather, there is a clear statistical correlation. Whether there is a causative relationship is an open question.)

YOU CANNOT AFFORD THE LUXURY OF FEAR, ANXIETY, ANGER, GUILT, OR DEPRESSION, NO MATTER WHAT THE CAUSE! AND YOU CAN'T AFFORD PREJUDICE, DISLIKE, HATRED, RESENTMENT, GREED, OR IGNORANCE. AT SOME LEVEL THERE HAS TO BE A PHYSIOLOGICAL NEGATIVE EFFECT.
—Norman Shealy

As I read about this research, I was driven to find out more about the connection between cancer, the mind, and emotions. I had a strong inner prompting that my own psychology had played a part in my illness. I knew that cancer does not grow overnight. Some experts estimate that it exists microscopically and slowly grows for up to five years before it is discovered. I began to wonder about the kind of "soil" that I had provided that had allowed the cancer to grow in my body. I knew in my heart that it was an important issue for me to resolve. Fortunately I had a very good therapist to assist me with this aspect of my healing. Dr. Marilyn Barrick helped me to be objective about my illness and also to get in touch with my feelings.

Like almost anyone diagnosed with a serious illness, I went through various emotions that follow a well-known pattern—shock, denial, anger, depression, acceptance. I also had to deal with a sense of guilt about getting the illness in the first place—here I was, a doctor and a minister who dealt with spiritual issues, and I had breast cancer. How could I have let this happen to me? Couldn't I see it coming?

Marilyn made it clear that guilt, shame, fear, anger, and bitterness are common emotions for many cancer patients, and they must be looked at and dealt with. Although many of these feelings are short-lived, if you don't acknowledge them and deal with them as they come up, they can simmer for a long time beneath the surface, eventually coloring your entire outlook on life and compromising your immune system.

I faced all of these emotions at some time during my treatment, and being able to talk about them and understand them with Marilyn's help was healing. We also worked on past emotions and my underlying psychology. Many people find inner child work is helpful in dealing with mental and emotional patterns that originate early in life.

I was acutely aware that I had daily choices to make about how I would react to the illness itself. I recall one day feeling how easy it would be to fall into a state of bitterness, so I immediately prayed and asked that all traces of this be removed. I could feel it leave me before it had a chance to take hold, and I can only imagine the angels coming to take the hardness of heart, bitterness, and resentment from me.

In addition to working with a therapist, I worked with my psychology on a spiritual level through prayer and other means. I asked the masters and angels of healing to work with Marilyn and me to help me deal with the emotional and psychological aspects of the cancer.

Is There a Cancer-Prone Personality?

There have long been theories of a link between cancer and the emotions. This connection, particularly with the emotions of grief and hopelessness, was described in the medical literature dating back to the nineteenth century. Yet somehow, the connection was forgotten in the mid–twentieth century as scientific advances seemed to offer the hope of treating cancer as a more localized condition.

Although almost everyone agrees that it is beneficial for cancer patients to work with their emotions, there has been much controversy about the subject of a "cancer-prone personality." It is said that people who have cancer or who are prone to cancer have a tendency to not express anger, to suppress or even "stuff" their emotions and to be overly compliant. Bernie Siegel and Lawrence LeShan have commented on the sense of hopelessness apparent in many cancer patients even before their condition was diagnosed, noting that cancer has also been linked to grief and deep sadness or sense of loss. It is thought that these and related emotions depress immunity and allow the growth of cancer.[7]

Many doctors are understandably opposed to the concept of a cancer-prone personality or that a cancer patient may be responsible for causing his or her cancer. They do not want their patients to subject themselves to needless blame or guilt. (And of course, if negative emotions lead to an increased risk of cancer, increasing guilt isn't likely to help.) Many, such as Dr. John Link, believe that "one's choices are not responsible for breast cancer."[8]

Andrew Weil, expert on mind-body medicine, states: "Health professionals who see a lot of cancer patients often describe them as 'nice'—that is, pleasant, inoffensive, unwilling to make trouble, apologetic for being sick. This frequent observation has given rise to the notion of a 'cancer personality.' In many ways it is just the opposite of the heart-attack personality with its tendency to rage."[9] Although Dr. Weil says that "it is reasonable to assume that living with a lot of unexpressed or unfelt grief and anger doesn't do you or your immune system any good," he believes that until further research is done, the concept of a cancer-prone personality is nothing more than an interesting idea.[10]

I also understand that blame and guilt are not helpful emotions, yet I do believe that my choices have an impact in my life and health. I see that as my accountability, without a sense of blame or guilt. I have a choice as to how I react to life's circumstances, and as I looked back on my life, following my diagnosis, I could see that I had made poor choices in some areas.

I think it is natural for a cancer patient to ask "why?" You want to examine your life to see if changes can be made and you want to find out what you can do to help overcome the condition. As I did this, I realized that if I were honest with myself, I could not lightly dismiss the traits of the cancer-prone personality that I could see clearly in myself—and I could not wait for the connection to be proven scientifically before beginning to work on correcting them.

Interestingly, if there were one word to describe my pre-cancer personality, it would have to be "nice." All my life, I have been described as a "nice" person, and I worked hard to be thought of that way. I even used to joke with my husband, Peter, about the "nice Neroli"—the face I showed to the world—and the "not-so-nice" or "naughty Neroli" who would pop up occasionally, though hardly ever in public. I usually complied with the wishes of other people, avoided confrontations, tended to swallow my emotions rather than express them, and went out of my way to help others—even to my own detriment. Now that I had breast cancer, I knew that I needed to change, and I had to find out more about the subject.

For anyone wanting to explore this path, a great place to start is *Cancer as a Turning Point*, a groundbreaking book by psychotherapist Lawrence LeShan, in which he reviews thirty-five years of mind-body medicine and speaks from his many years of experience with cancer patients. His book is excellent reading for any cancer patient and reveals that the subject of the cancer-prone personality is not a trivial or simple one.

Dr. LeShan says, "The best of the new research that has appeared in recent years has presented results pointing out that psychological factors do play a part in how and when people become sick and how their immune systems function when they are sick. Psychological factors are certainly only one part of the process—no one 'makes themselves sick' by how they behave or feel. Other factors such as heredity and the physical environment play a major role as well. *You are not responsible for becoming ill, and you are not responsible for your recovery.* What you *are* responsible for once you are ill is to do your best to get better. This means getting the best medical treatment possible *and* changing your life so that your inner healing abilities will be stimulated to the highest level possible."[11]

Dr. LeShan speaks of patients who deal with cancer on all three levels of human life—physical, psychological, and spiritual. After years of working with cancer patients, he has found that those who consciously work on all three levels tend to do better than those who do not.[12]

He also believes that the big changes happen *inside* and not outside the patient. "The inside is the important and crucial place that change needs to take place if we are trying to move our immune system to higher levels of functioning. Changes in the outer life may or may not occur, they may be dramatic when they do, but they are reflections of our inner change."[13]

Dr. LeShan notes that cancer-prone individuals often show the traits of passivity, despair, and suppression of emotional expression. Although not all of these traits applied to me, there were elements of all of them in me. Much of what Dr. LeShan said in his book resonated deeply within me.

At the end of his book is a series of exercises designed to help patients contact their inner self, the desires and wants and hopes that have been suppressed in the desire to conform to the expectations of others. Dr. LeShan found that as patients worked through these exercises and tapped the unexpressed potential of the soul and spirit, the inner resources of the physical body would also be activated. It was amazing to read the stories of terminal cancer patients whose tumors would spontaneously start to shrink once they found their real purpose in life and began to live it. As I worked through the exercises, I gained new insight into my life and the choices I made each day.

Even more telling than Dr. LeShan's description of character traits was the discussion of stress and how people deal with problems in life. I remembered the words I had read some years earlier: "The most important part of any experience you have is not what is flung your way but your reaction to it."[14] I could see that although there were situations in my life that were beyond my control, I could have handled my reaction to them much better. I did not have to see myself as a victim.

This was one of the most important things that I worked on with my psychologist. I also worked on this with Bach Flower Remedies, homeopathy, and essential oils. Here is where I believe that I made some of my greatest personal progress. It has changed the way that I think about myself and how I approach my life today.

THE SYMBOLISM OF BREAST CANCER

Louise Hay is a best-selling author and metaphysical lecturer who has taught for many years on the connection between the mind and emotions and physical illness. In her book *Heal Your Body: The Mental Causes for Physical Illness and the Metaphysical Way to Overcome Them,* she interprets the breast as representing "mothering and nurturing and nourishment." She considers breast problems to be related to "a refusal to nourish the self. Putting everyone else first. Overmothering. Overprotection. Overbearing attitude." She interprets cancer as related to "Deep hurt. Long-standing resentment. Deep secret or grief eating away at the self."[15]

Hay believes that a primary cause of disease is unhealthy mental patterns such as these and that changing these mental patterns can be a powerful means of healing. One tool that she teaches for reprogramming the mind is the use of affirmations—positive statements about the self that are repeated many times a day. She offers two affirmations for breast cancer which I said daily for some time:

> *I take in and give out nourishment in perfect balance.*
> *I lovingly forgive and release all of the past. I choose to fill my world with joy. I love and approve of myself.* [16]

SETTING BOUNDARIES

In the physical body, it is the assignment of the immune system to set boundaries. It decides what is and is not "you" and then takes care of those things that are not you that somehow got into the body. Cancer can only grow if the immune system doesn't recognize this growth as something that should not be there, and many complementary cancer therapies are intended to activate and strengthen the immune system rather than attack cancer cells directly.

There is a great deal of research now to show how the mind-body connection influences the immune system. In *Love, Medicine, and Miracles*, Bernie Siegel refers to a follow-up study in the *New England Journal of Medicine* of fifty-seven women with early breast cancer. The study showed that "recurrence-free survival was significantly commoner among patients who reacted to cancer with denial or 'fighting spirit' than among patients who responded with stoic acceptance or feelings of helplessness or hopelessness."[17] Lower survival rates from cancer are associated with depression or helplessness, and higher rates are associated with a sense of coping. The personality traits of a sense of meaning and purpose in life, a sense of personal responsibility for one's health, an ability to express one's needs and emotions, and a sense of humor all enhance survival. Conversely, "compliance, conformity, self-sacrifice, denial of hostility or anger, and non-expression of emotion" seem to be related to an unfavorable prognosis in cancer patients and may possibly relate to susceptibility to cancer as well.[18]

LOWER SURVIVAL RATES FROM CANCER ARE ASSOCIATED WITH DEPRESSION OR HELPLESSNESS, AND HIGHER RATES ARE ASSOCIATED WITH A SENSE OF COPING.

What we learn from these studies is that people who have a strong sense of self—who know what they want and go for it—have better outcomes. As I was reading about these patterns and at the same time working on strengthening my immune system to deal with the cancer, I realized that there were clear parallels and that one way of looking at the profile of patients who do well is that they have healthy immune systems on mental and emotional levels.

What would a healthy "mental immune system" look like? As it is with the physical, it is knowing what is you and what is not you. It is knowing what your thoughts are versus what is seeking to enter your mind from the outside. One source of these outside influences is the media, which constantly bombards us, telling us what we should think about every issue or topic. It constantly tries to shape how we think about the world and about ourselves.

What do we think about ourselves? Do we allow the condemnation of the world to enter: the messages that we are too fat, not pretty enough, not intelligent enough? Do we accept thoughts of depression and gloom? We can internalize all of this negativity if we are too passive and take things in without discrimination.

We must also be mindful of the messages we internalize from friends, family, and coworkers. The things we internalize in childhood go especially deep; they can become an integral part of who we are and how we see ourselves. Our task is to separate ourselves from others' concepts of us. Although it may be painful, this process can be tremendously liberating and a key to finding out who we really are and what our purpose in life is.

What about the "emotional immune system"? How am I to know what is "me" (my wants and desires) and what is "not me" (what everybody else wants me to do)? As I thought about this, I realized that I put a lot of energy into doing what other people wanted me to do—or what I *thought* they wanted me to do. Sometimes I was so concerned with making other people happy that I no longer even really knew what I wanted to do.

Many of the exercises in Dr. LeShan's book are designed to help you get back in touch with your inner desires. Your soul has come to earth with a mission to fulfill. This sense of mission and purpose can get buried under the desires of friends, family, and loved ones. How many people do we see who become doctors or lawyers because their parents wanted them to? Then they get to middle age and experience the classic mid-life crisis, realizing that they have taken a detour from their soul's intended route.

Sometimes the crisis is brought on by illness such as breast cancer. I know that as soon as I heard the diagnosis, everything shifted. Suddenly I knew that I had to do what was most important to me, and I could no longer keep doing things simply because other people expected or wanted me to do them.

This was not an easy task—sometimes the inner desires of the soul get so deeply buried that it is hard to even find them again. However, Marilyn and others helped me to get in touch with my "real self." Although I am essentially the same "nice Neroli," there is a big difference in my post-breast-cancer personality. I don't automatically do what other people want when their wishes conflict with my own. I no longer have such an aversion to saying no when I think it is the right thing to do. I am more willing to speak my mind when it is appropriate and I am generally less passive.

I am still devoted to service and helping others, but I can set better boundaries now and consciously decide whether or not I will involve myself in a particular situation. If I do, it is my choice and not another's. Although I still like to work hard at a job that I love, I am more able to take time for myself.

I have found as a consequence that I am not so universally liked—sometimes when I say no, people get upset. But that is a part of the price that I pay to be true to myself and follow my heart. It is worth it to me.

What I am saying here is true for me, yet I know it may not be true for everyone. I have known many breast-cancer patients who fit this profile—and also a number who do not. Nevertheless, I believe that if you have any form of cancer and you want to look into this area of your life, it can pay big dividends. However, it has to be your own "want" and not something that is forced upon you by others. (After all, if you're working on your psychology merely because someone else thinks you should, you are still living someone else's life and not your own.)

In general, I believe that it is better that patients discover these things for themselves. If their soul wants to know, they will ask the questions and seek the answers. I looked at these things because I had a burning drive to do so. For others, it may be of no interest at all. And that's fine too.

Bernie Siegel says, "Everyone can be an exceptional patient, and the best time to start is before getting sick. Many people don't make full use of their life force until a near-fatal illness goads them into a 'change of mind.' But it doesn't have to be a last-minute awakening. The mind's power is available to us all the time, and it has more room to maneuver before disaster threatens. This process doesn't require allegiance to any particular religious belief or psychological system."[19]

A Mental and Emotional Diet

As well as learning to set boundaries mentally and emotionally, I also had to think about my mental and emotional diet. We are learning more and more about what to feed our body. But what do we feed our mind?

It has been said, "As a man thinketh in his heart, so is he."[20] Our thoughts are things, and they have a profound effect on our body, mind, and soul. As we observe the mind, we soon realize that what we take in as food for the mind makes a difference. The kinds of programs we watch on television, the kinds of conversations we have, the books we read, the movies we see, the places we go—all of these things affect our thoughts. Some of these effects happen very quickly and can be easily recorded in medical tests. Some of them can have long-term effects as they shape our thought processes and our overall outlook on life.

While I was sick, I learned to be more and more selective. I became careful of the things I put into my mind, for I often found them surfacing in the middle of the night. I deliberately sought out uplifting movies, books, and magazines. I spent time in nature and with uplifting friends, and I chose my friends more carefully. I worked on forgiveness so that I would have no additional baggage to carry around. I also worked on freeing my thoughts from criticism of myself and others. It is so easy to judge and condemn others, and often we are most critical of ourselves.

DREAMS AND HEALING

Several times in my life, I have had dreams that contained a special message. These dreams had an entirely different quality from other dreams. They were very vivid and "real." I always had a sense that there was an important meaning in them. Sometimes the message would be clear, and sometimes it was in symbols that needed to be decoded. Shortly after the diagnosis of breast cancer I began to have a series of very significant dreams that proved to be beneficial in a number of ways once I understood them.

The close correspondence between physical illness and the content of dreams is a concept that goes back a long way. Hippocrates thought that some dreams had the potential to indicate diseases and physical conditions. Aristotle wrote, "The beginnings of diseases and other distempers which are about to visit the body ... must be more evident in the sleeping than in the waking state."[21] In more recent times, therapists and authors have written about dreams, dream analysis, and dream interpretation. Freud said that dreams were the "royal road" to the unconscious.

A number of researchers today believe that dreams may be helpful in diagnosing illness. They provide a window into the subconscious and a means of communication between the body and the mind. Dream researcher Robert Van de Castle explains that in some cases dreams can almost seem to serve as X-rays, giving very specific information about illness and often predating the appearance of physical symptoms or other signs of the illness.[22] He gives many examples of dreams that have heralded the onset of physical illness in his book *Our Dreaming Mind.*

Bernie Siegel describes dreams as messages from the unconscious that can be interpreted at two levels. The first is at the level of "personal meanings." He says that this can almost always be worked out in discussion with the patient and that almost anyone can understand the personal meaning of dreams if they take the time to apply some basic principles and if they talk about their dreams. The second is the "deeper, unconscious level of symbols and myths, which is more problematic" and difficult to interpret.[23]

I approached my dreams at both levels and gained many important insights. As far as I am aware, I did not have any dreams that gave a premonition of my cancer, but on two occasions significant dreams helped me to confirm a course of medical treatment and enabled me to take actions that were necessary to my healing.

The first dream happened soon after my second surgery, which was to sample some of the lymph nodes in my armpit to see if they contained cancerous cells. It occurred when I was back home, some days after I had recovered from this operation. I was in the midst of deciding whether to go ahead with chemotherapy, and I was mentally preparing myself for it. I want to stress that this was not just an ordinary dream. It was almost a waking dream—very vivid. On the night of February 24, I dreamed that I was shown that three of the seven lymph nodes were cancerous. There was no fear in the dream, but it was clear that I needed to know the information.

When I awoke, I knew its meaning. While I was happy that the medical pathology revealed that the nodes were negative on the macroscopic or physical level, the dream gave an insight on a deeper level—perhaps that cancer cells had already spread microscopically, or that this existed as a potential. This awareness helped me make the difficult decision to go ahead with the chemotherapy. It confirmed my intuition that the cancer was more serious than the test showed. I felt that the prayer and spiritual work that I and my friends were doing was making a difference and holding the disease at bay. And while I trusted the spiritual work, I also got the message that this was a serious situation and that I had to do everything that I could to arrest the cancer at all levels. Chemotherapy was not my preference, but I felt compelled to go forward with it in order to leave no stone unturned.

The next dream occurred about a month later, when I had already begun chemotherapy—which was a scary thing for me to do to my body, knowing of the potential side effects. On the evening of my first day of the chemotherapy, I went to sleep, very concerned over whether I had done the right thing, and I had another vivid dream.

I dreamed that I was standing at the top of a huge cliff with my husband, Peter. He was dressed in flowing Oriental robes in brilliant colors of green, blue, and purple—colors I associated with healing. He began instructing me and was writing in Chinese symbols on a wall a little way back from the top of the cliff. He indicated that I should dive off the cliff into the deep, dark blue waters below. He was not asking or directing me, but telling me that I had that option. I was very afraid and reluctant, but he told me that if I chose to dive, I would go very deep into the water, and then I would surface again.

With his reassurance, I dived off the cliff. It was indeed a long way down before I finally hit the water. I went down deep into the water and eventually swam up to the surface. Later in the dream, I met a friend from Australia, and we walked hand in hand along the beach. I said to her, "Did you know that I had breast cancer?" She said that she did know, and then the dream ended.

Chemotherapy certainly felt like that dive off the cliff to me. It was very scary, but the dream told me that although it would be intense and potentially dangerous, I would make it and resurface in the end. It helped me to keep going, and I would often recall that dream when the chemotherapy became intense. I also noted in the dream that I told my friend that I "had" cancer (past tense). In other words, after the dive into the water (the chemotherapy), I would no longer have cancer.

There were other dreams—too personal to share here—that taught me lessons about what the illness of cancer meant from a spiritual and emotional standpoint. My therapist was particularly helpful in discerning the meaning of these dreams. To me, the importance of the right therapist cannot be overestimated. Although I was often on the right track, I am not sure that I could have unraveled all the intricacies of my dreams without Marilyn Barrick's help.

Working with Your Therapist

If you decide to use the services of a therapist, it is important to choose one who is right for you. Dr. LeShan recommends taking the time to do this and suggests this method of finding a therapist: "Find the experienced and seasoned therapists in your area. Ask the local medical society and the local psychological association. Assuming that they are trained people, start a shopping procedure. See them one at a time until you find one that you like—someone with whom the chemistry is good and whom you would like to have as a friend. You may have to see a number of them. That is the first essential. Unless there is a liking, you may get somewhere, but it will take you nine times as long and be nine times as hard."[24]

I agree with his assessment. I was fortunate to have Marilyn nearby. She was able to combine work with my dreams with psychotherapy. Often I knew when it was time to see her again, because another dream would surface. She also had a deep understanding of the spiritual life and the role of the heaven-world in the life of the soul.

My answer to those who ask how to find the right therapist would be to seek higher assistance from the beginning. Ask heaven for guidance—your Higher Self or guardian angel can lead you to the right person. If you follow your heart, and any little leads that your Higher Self might send, it is amazing where it can lead you. This simple process works—ask and ye shall receive.

Once you have found the right therapist (or the best possible one), ask the heaven-world to overshadow and work through that therapist. Here is a simple technique that I have often used. You have a Higher Self and a guardian angel, and so does your doctor, surgeon, oncologist, therapist—in fact, anyone you are working with for healing. The night before any meeting with those involved in your care—especially any meetings that you expect may be difficult—call for the guardian angel and the Higher Self of everyone involved, including yourself, to meet in the heavenly retreats while everyone is sleeping.

In this way, everything can be worked out in the heaven-world ahead of time, and everyone will be totally prepared and able to discuss things when you meet in the physical. When you sit down to have the meeting the next day, simply acknowledge inwardly the presence of the guardian angel and the Higher Self of each person in the room.

It is a simple technique, but I have seen it work in many areas of life—business meetings, meetings with lawyers, meetings with family members, counseling sessions—in fact, any situation of importance.

THE HEALING POWER OF MUSIC

The healing effects of sound and music on the human mind and body are profound and well documented. Many mind-body programs include music as a technique to activate the body's natural powers of healing.

There is a lot we do not know about music and its effects on the body, but, as Michael Castleman explains, we do know some of the mechanisms by which music helps in healing: "At least some of its therapeutic power comes from its ability to trigger the release of endorphins, the powerful opiate-like chemicals produced in the brain that induce euphoria and reduce pain.... [Music] reduces levels of stress hormones such as adrenaline. It has a calming effect on the limbic system, a group of structures within the brain that regulates emotions. And it boosts levels of immunoglobulin A (IgA), the body's first line of defense against colds and other infections."[25]

I have always noted the calming effect of classical music, so it was natural for me to utilize music in my healing journey. I began each day by listening to a favorite piece of music, "Pomp and Circumstance," by Elgar. I took it with me each time I traveled to chemotherapy. As I played the piece, I meditated and composed prayers that captured my life's desires. At times I would get clear inner direction as to what I needed to do next.

Music quickly became a soothing, comforting, and often uplifting part of the day. I listened several times to Andrew Weil's production, *Sound Body, Sound Mind*. It contains instruction on the effects of music and a sixty-minute piece of music specifically designed for healing.

During my treatment, a friend sent me a newspaper clipping of an article from the *Chicago Tribune* titled "The Healing Power of Harps." It told the story of a group of people led by Ronald Price, who holds a Ph.D. in special education and whose own cerebral-palsy symptoms remained in remission as long as he played the harp every day. As a professor, he began a research project in harp-music therapy because he wanted to see whether the remarkable healing effect he had experienced could be replicated in others with neurological disorders. Dr. Price now plays the harp for patients and sees its powerful healing effects on people of all ages.[26]

Some music has the ability to take you to other dimensions of your being and to allow you to access areas of yourself that you might not be expressing or using. These dimensions are spheres of consciousness of your own Higher Self. When I was young, my father taught me something of this aspect of music. A favorite uncle of mine was deaf almost from birth, and although he could not hear with his outer ears, he often heard beautiful, unearthly music with his "inner hearing." My father explained to him that he was not imagining this heavenly music—he was hearing the music of the spheres.

Some of the great musicians and composers have been able to capture elements of this music. For example, Beethoven composed some of his greatest works at the end of his life, when he was deaf. He could no longer hear the sounds of this world, but he was able to bring back sounds from other spheres and compose music that can take us to other planes of consciousness.

I tried to find music that captured this quality—music that could take me outside of my day-to-day thought and feeling processes and to a higher dimension of being. I found that this music could help me forget the details of my treatment, allowing me to focus on the light that would be the real source of my healing.

I used gentle and relaxing classical music as a background for my exercise. I walked to classical music. I sat in the hot springs and absorbed its healing sound. Besides classical music of the great composers, at various times I listened to Gregorian chants, sacred Christmas music, Russian choral works, Eastern music, Indian music, including the classical *bhajans*, and Tibetan Buddhist mantras.

LAUGHTER, THE BEST MEDICINE

Finally, I believe that humor is essential to healing. Norman Cousins, author of the classic best-seller *Anatomy of an Illness as Perceived by the Patient,* attributed his healing from the crippling disease ankylosing spondylitis to "humor therapy." He watched Marx Brothers movies and others that made him laugh, and he found that if he laughed for ten minutes, he was able to get two hours of pain-free, uninterrupted sleep.

I was often amazed that if you get a group of recovering cancer patients together, sooner or later they start telling stories and eventually get around to laughing. Some of us who stayed together while we went through treatment enjoyed getting together and laughing at ourselves. I can remember one hilarious session when we tried on all kinds of wigs and hats that we were or had been using during chemotherapy.

Peter made it his job to keep me from becoming too serious, which is one of my traits. He could often catch me off guard and make me laugh at myself or the situation that I was in. One day, we rented a bunch of funny movies and sat down to watch them in order to get the endorphins going. Although not all of them were funny to us, and some actually made us cry, it all helped.

Laughter truly is great medicine and can actually ease pain, both emotional and physical.

Journal Entry
February 13, 1999
Five questions from Bernie Siegel for cancer patients: [27]

1. Do you want to live to be a hundred?

Not sure, maybe. If I do, I have to learn not to worry, to live each day as it comes, and to live in a more full and loving way, to depend more on God and less upon my human self.

2. What happened in the year or two before your illness?

As I look back I feel that I had two awful years—they were painful and agonizing. I felt forced into a cramped space with no room to move. I changed jobs several times and went through big changes in my life at all levels.

3. Why do you need your illness and what benefits do you derive from it?

I feel that I escaped from the cramped conditions. The illness got me out gracefully and gave me permission and time to mend, to heal, to learn, to live, to love. It gives me opportunity to pause and rest. It stopped me literally from "killing myself." It changes my whole direction.

4. What does the illness mean to you?

The illness means an initiation or testing of the heart—it is teaching me to allow my heart to open more. I am aware that it also means, "Physician, heal thyself." I must do all that I can do to heal myself. I am no longer the caretaker of others but now must allow others to care for me, as they will. I can rest and sleep and "be."
I can forgive and let go of hardness of heart and resentment. I am not responsible for others. I do not need to sacrifice myself for others to the exclusion of caring for myself. I can now look cancer in the face and overcome any fear of death as the last enemy.

5. Describe your disease and what you are experiencing.

Cancer is a turning point in my life. Everything changes. I am reexamining everything. There are many benefits to this disease. It is hard, but in some ways I feel that I have been rescued from myself. I am taking better care of myself. I am now getting more rest and taking time for relaxation. In a strange way I am experiencing less stress. I am very focused on getting well. I am sleeping a lot. I am learning to overcome fear. I am feeling more love, more loved, and more loving. I have let go of a number of attachments that were harmful. I have changed my diet, my exercise habits, and my outlook. I have learned to say no in a big way. There are some things that I will no longer do and will not go back to.

CHECKLIST: WORKING WITH THE MIND AND EMOTIONS

✓ Get the best medical treatment possible—and also change your life so that your inner healing power will be unleashed.

✓ Assess yourself objectively.

✓ Involve a Higher Power in your life—by whatever name you call it.

✓ Ask to be shown the areas of your life that need change.

✓ Watch your thoughts. Weed out the unhelpful ones.

✓ Get expert help to deal with emotions.

✓ Work with a therapist or psychologist. Ask your Higher Self or guardian angel to lead you to the right person.

✓ Avoid blame and guilt.

✓ Live your life—not someone else's.

✓ Find your mission and start living it.

✓ Love yourself and be kind to yourself.

✓ Learn to set loving boundaries—mentally, emotionally and physically.

✓ Remember that you are a work in progress. Don't be hard on yourself if you make some mistakes.

✓ Send your body "live" messages.

✓ Harness the power of your imagination.

    o Visualize healthy immune cells dissolving the cancer cells
    o Visualize healing colors:
       ▪ Violet for change and transformation
       ▪ Green for healing
       ▪ Blue for protection and alignment with the divine plan

✓ Pay attention to your dreams and the messages that they send to you from your subconscious.

✓ Use the healing power of music.

✓ Activate your sense of humor—it can boost your immune system.

CHAPTER 14

SPIRITUALITY AND HEALING

I knew almost from the beginning that in my journey through cancer I would have to pursue healing spiritually as well as on physical, emotional, and mental levels. I used many spiritual healing techniques to help my body to fight the cancer, to get my body back into balance, and to boost my immune system. For me this was not just something that I did "as well as"—it was a key part of the program.

I was diligent in my spiritual work and took time every day for my spiritual practice. As well as all the other benefits, this helped me to feel that I was doing some of the work and not just leaving it all to chance or luck or the doctors and their treatments.

HEALING PRAYER

Prayer has always been a part of my life, but once the diagnosis was made, I prayed with renewed vigor and determination—and also with more love.

In addition to my own prayer, there were many others who prayed for me from the time I had the mammogram until the end of my radiotherapy. I would tell everyone whom I met and who asked after me, "Please pray for me." It was one way to surrender myself into God's hands and ask others for help, which was in itself an important part of my journey.

In fact, much of my prayer was to commend my spirit to God and surrender the outcome to him, even as I asked to be healed. There comes a time when you just have to commit yourself to God's care and ask him to take care of all the details—whether you live or die, or if you live, what kind of life you will lead. Our lives are a gift, and it is by his grace that we live. Even though you may have offered such prayers many times in your life, I can assure you that prayer takes on new meaning when you are given a diagnosis of cancer and have to face all that the word *cancer* entails.

My name was on a number of prayer lists from America to Russia to Australia. An aunt in Australia put my name in her local Catholic prayer group. A friend, a practitioner of the Baha'i faith, prayed for me, and many family members, friends, and coworkers joined me in prayer. When I went to the hospital for treatments, I filled out prayer request slips that I put in the boxes they had provided for that purpose. The hospital staff would also pray for me, and with me, if I asked.

I am not alone in the desire for healing prayer. Studies show that 75 percent of us believe that doctors should address spiritual issues as a part of medical care, and 50 percent would like their doctors to pray not just for them, but with them.[1]

Science is just now catching up with what many people have known for years. The person who has probably done the most to promote the scientific study of prayer in healing is Larry Dossey. Initially a skeptic, he came across scientific studies documenting the effectiveness of prayer and eventually came to the conclusion that he had to be willing to look at the facts, even though they did not fit with his preconceived ideas. He felt that he could not ignore the evidence without feeling like "a traitor to the scientific tradition."[2]

In his book *Prayer is Good Medicine,* Dr. Dossey says, "Prayer is back. After sitting on the sidelines for most of this century, prayer is moving towards center stage in modern medicine. Doctors are taking prayer not just into their offices, clinics, and hospitals, but into experimental laboratories as well."[3] And they are getting results.

Statistically speaking, prayer is effective. More and more controlled laboratory experiments show that prayer can bring about measurable changes. Dossey covers the subject of prayer and healing thoroughly and from a scientific standpoint, and his three books include results from many scientific studies.

He quotes one widely-publicized experiment by cardiologist Randolph Byrd, which showed that patients in a coronary-care unit who were prayed for did significantly better than those who were not prayed for. They had fewer complications and needed less medication. Dossey commented on this study, "If the technique being studied had been a new drug or a surgical procedure instead of prayer, it would almost certainly have been heralded as some sort of 'breakthrough.'"[4]

Scientists have proven that prayer is effective. But perhaps the reason they are not heralding it as a breakthrough is that science today is less comfortable talking about how and why it works. It is as if a wall has been erected between science and spirituality—but it is a wall that is entirely artificial, created by man and not by God. We have to be willing to break down the wall (or at least peep over the top) if we want to really understand life, or even the world around us.

Prayer is the language of the soul. In its essence, it is simply conversation with God—communion with him and listening to his answers. Dr. Dossey says that a key factor in the effectiveness of prayer seems to be the love that accompanies it. The particular religion of the prayer or the person who prays does not seem to matter. This reminds me of my father's likening the spiritual path to climbers taking different routes up a mountain but all eventually arriving at the same destination at the top. It is not your religion or lack of it; it is the love in your heart that produces change.

Was I surprised by these results? Not at all. Although I was glad to see science catching up with spirituality, I had always believed in the effectiveness of prayer and had seen its results many times in my life and in the lives of my patients.

If I had to quantify it, as impossible as it would be to do, I would guess that prayer (mine and others) and spiritual practice was at least 50 percent of the reason that I recovered and did so well during my treatment. When I get to heaven, I may find that 50 percent was a conservative estimate—maybe prayer was 75 percent. Or maybe I will find that other things contributed more than I realized. However, I do know that prayer was a mainstay of my treatment. It was the framework upon which everything else hung.

At times I was lifted up by the prayers and good wishes of people who I knew were praying for me. It was a real boost to meet people who would say, "You are in my prayers!" Sometimes it was people in my church or community whom I barely knew, and I was so grateful. The knowledge that people cared for me helped me to feel good about myself on the not-so-good days and often brought tears to my eyes.

I was especially grateful for the prayers of my spiritual teacher, Elizabeth Clare Prophet. I could feel the light and the energy that she radiated to me as she prayed for me by phone each day for more than two weeks.

I am sure that heartfelt prayer reduced the size of the tumor from two centimeters on the mammogram and ultrasound to one centimeter at biopsy three days later. I think that it was also due to prayer that the lymph nodes were clear in the biopsy, which pushed my diagnosis from stage II to stage I. My medical mind tells me that most doctors would be very skeptical about this, and of course, I have no way of proving it. Nevertheless, I believe in my heart that it is true.

SCIENTIFIC PRAYER

Just as physical scientists are discovering the power of prayer, spiritual teachers have always known that there are scientific methods of prayer.

The beloved Indian saint and yogi Paramahansa Yogananda taught that the first rule of prayer is to approach God only with legitimate desires. The second is to pray for their fulfillment not as a beggar but as a son of God the Father. He said, "Be practical and earnest about prayer. Concentrate deeply on what you are praying."[5]

There was a special group of about ten close friends around the country whose help I enlisted for this kind of prayer. These were people who knew how to pray scientifically and combine prayer with focused visualizations. I would e-mail them a few days before my treatment and tell them what was happening with me and the details of my treatment. I would also tell them what visualizations I was using, and they would often e-mail back with suggestions and refinements that were extremely helpful.

BE PRACTICAL AND EARNEST ABOUT PRAYER.

CONCENTRATE DEEPLY ON WHAT YOU ARE PRAYING.

—Yogananda

For example, I would tell them to pray that the chemotherapy only go where it was intended to go in my body, that it not damage any healthy cells, and that my white-cell counts and blood counts would not be reduced (or would be reduced just enough so that the doctors could see that the chemotherapy was working and not want to increase the dosage unnecessarily). I also asked them to pray that I would not have nausea, hair loss, mouth ulcers, diarrhea, or other unwanted side effects. After each treatment I would let them know how it went and we would refine our visualizations.

I combined my own prayers with the visualizations I mentioned earlier in the book. I visualized violet light and healing green light entering my body and dissolving the cancer, restoring everything to its original, divine order. During chemotherapy, at the suggestion of one of my prayer partners, I used the blue and the violet colors in particular—the blue for protection of the healthy cells in my body and the violet for change and transformation where it was needed.

Sometimes I worked at the visualization on a cellular level, seeing the cancer cells being dissolved and removed by my healthy immune system. At other times I held a more general visualization and allowed my body to work out the details.

THE POWER OF THE SPOKEN WORD

One form of prayer that I used a great deal was to recite mantras to invite the light into my body. In the East, people repeat mantras over and over, many times a day. In the West, we are not as accustomed to this practice. However, each time you repeat a prayer or a mantra, you strengthen its power by investing it with more and more of the light and energy of God that is flowing through you.

The benefits of repeated prayer and mantra have been known by mystics for centuries. Many have reported having transcendent experiences using this practice. They have achieved profound changes in their lives—spiritual and even physical.

Scientists in the West are now discovering the power of mantra. In the early 1970s, Dr. Herbert Benson, president and founder of the Mind/Body Medical Institute at Harvard Medical School, documented a phenomenon he dubbed the "relaxation response," which he says is the opposite of the body's fight-or-flight mechanism.

In his experiments, Bensen told his subjects to sit quietly, repeat a Sanskrit mantra mentally or verbally for ten to twenty minutes, breathe regularly, and push intruding thoughts aside. He found that those who repeated a mantra for as little as ten minutes a day experienced measurable physiological changes, including reduced heart rate, lower stress levels, and slower metabolism. Those with high blood pressure lowered their blood pressure. These changes did not occur just while they were saying the mantra but lasted throughout the day. Subsequent studies have shown that repeating mantras can benefit the immune system, relieve insomnia, and reduce the need for visits to the doctor.[6]

Bensen found that other words or phrases had the same effect. Even words like one, ocean, love, and peace produced the response. It appears that there is a universal principle at work here: the practice allows human beings to enter a different physiological state.

However, beyond the physiological changes that Bensen documented, there are also spiritual benefits. More subjective and thus more difficult to document scientifically, they are just as important—perhaps more so. Many people find that repetition of mantras allows the mind to focus on God. Whether it is Buddhists reciting their mantras, Orthodox monks reciting the Jesus Prayer, or Christians reciting the rosary, they find a sense of peace and oneness with God through the repetition of spoken prayer. And I have found this to be true in my own life.

REPEATING MANTRAS CAN BENEFIT THE IMMUNE SYSTEM, RELIEVE INSOMNIA, AND REDUCE THE NEED FOR VISITS TO THE DOCTOR.

Devotion is the key to the power of mantra, song, and prayer. You can use any mantra that appeals to you and that is sponsored by a being in heaven. You may want to give the rosary to Mary, recite Buddhist mantras, offer Christian prayers or Jewish devotions, or sing the sacred Hindu chants known as bhajans. Do whatever means the most to you and whatever activates that power of devotion and love within you.

I gave all of the above. I gave prayers to Archangel Michael for protection. I prayed to Archangel Raphael and Mary for healing. I was, and still am, devoted to the rosary, and I gave it every day of my treatment. In choosing to pray, you really can't go wrong. Prayer is the cheapest form of treatment that there is.

Mantras, in particular, helped me to find peace and greater contact with my Higher Self during my treatment. One mantra was a favorite because it is easy to remember and say any time, even while doing other things. It is an affirmation of the violet light and the violet flame, which is known as a transformative energy that changes darkness into light, sickness into health, negative energy into a positive manifestation.

I AM a being of violet fire,
I AM the purity God desires.

The words "I AM" refer to the Higher Self, and the meaning of the affirmation is that "God within me is qualifying the energy flowing through me as violet fire. God is manifesting in me the purity that he desires."

I would repeat this and other mantras many times throughout the course of the day, sometimes with full devotion and concentration, even as a meditation. At other times I would give them while I was doing other things, such as cooking or driving. I even gave them in the shower as I visualized the violet light tinged with emerald green flowing over my body as the water came down around me. In a pool at the hot springs, I might visualize violet- or green-colored water and imagine that my body was soaking in its healing essence.

I have found prayer and mantra to be like the oil in the gears that makes the engine of life run smoothly. They sustained me through the difficult times and brought a greater light and joy to the good times. And I can never fully express my gratitude and appreciation for those who prayed and did spiritual work for me while I was dealing with the challenges of my journey through cancer.

MEDITATION

Meditation is another spiritual practice that is gaining increasing popularity, even within the medical community. In the early 1980s, Joan Borysenko and Herbert Benson cofounded a mind-body medical clinic under the auspices of the Harvard Medical School. The program was designed to teach patients how to boost their immune system, overcome chronic pain, and alleviate the symptoms of a host of stress-related illnesses through prayer, meditation, and other means.

Borysenko's national best seller *Minding the Body, Mending the Mind* describes various simple but effective meditation exercises. She says, "The primary goal of meditation is not relaxation—it is awareness. This is what eventually leads to getting the mind back under control. Relaxation is a side effect of learning how to meditate."[7] I particularly enjoyed reading about her self-expressed evolution from "worrier" to "warrior"—I could certainly relate!

There are many different forms of meditation. Some originate in Eastern spiritual practices. Some have evolved from the spiritual traditions of Christian and Jewish mystics. Others have been developed as simple exercises for the mind and do not have a spiritual background. The basic principle is to still the conscious mind and bring a peace and harmony to one's thought processes. Many people like to have something of a spiritual nature as their point of concentration and derive great benefit from this.

If you wish to pursue meditation, find a method that appeals to you and fits with your beliefs. Many people in the West who have grown up with the mass media (which trains people to have short attention spans) find that meditation combined with the saying of mantras or prayers works best. One good resource for meditation is Lawrence LeShan's little book, *How to Meditate*.

SPIRITUAL DIRECTION

Sometimes on my journey I would pray and ask God to give me specific direction or show me what I needed to know. When putting out a call to the universe in this way, it was amazing to see what came back on the return current. When I began to seek answers, the universe found ways of providing them.

These might take the form of something I came across in a magazine, something I saw by chance while flipping channels, something that happened to arrive in the mail at exactly the right time, or any of a myriad of amazing ways that the universe seems to be able to speak to us.

God does have ways of sending us signs, but it is also good to remember that not everything is a sign from "on high." It is not good to go too far with this and become superstitious about any little event that happens in your life. Prayer can help to discern the difference between true guidance and distractions that come from the mass consciousness or negative momentums in our own subconscious. I would always check these things out before acting on them, applying intuition and common sense. If something felt right in my heart, I would follow it. If it didn't, I would not.

One way these calls were answered was through good friends who always seemed to show up at the right time. Two weeks before chemo-therapy, I was actively looking for ways to make the chemotherapy more bearable. One of these friends had worked with herbs and natural heal-ing methods all her life, and we began one morning at breakfast talking about different herbs and what they could do.

We drove to Bozeman and went to a health food store, where we came across a book by a well-known herbalist. I bought the book, then we wandered through the aisles in a kind of prayerful reverie. We looked up the material that appealed to us in the book, flipping through the pages and finding a gem here and there. There was a great feeling of satisfaction as we took the products off the shelves and put them in the shopping basket. As we moved from aisle to aisle, I could feel the presence of angels. I had a joyous sense of the rightness of the herbs and tinctures that we chose.

After finishing at the health food store, we found an herbal shop that had just opened. I had read about burdock-root oil for prevention of hair loss during chemotherapy but could not find it on the shelves. I went to ask if they had any, and the owner of the store pointed to another woman at the counter who happened to be a clinical herbalist. She told me how to make the oil, using burdock root and olive oil. Later, she told me that she had helped her husband overcome cancer of the kidney using herbs. And so, through what seemed to be a coincidence, I was led to the herbalist who made the herbal tinctures that helped me through chemotherapy.

There were a couple of occasions when I did not follow these impulses and wished later that I had. Praying for direction is only half the story: you also have to be able to recognize an answer when it comes your way—and, of course, act on it. Part of the spiritual path is being open to finding answers anywhere and anytime.

THE IMAGE OF PERFECTION

I believe that the body is intended to be a temple for the indwelling Spirit. It is a vehicle for our evolution in the journey of life. We cannot become overly attached to it or become slaves to its needs—one day we will lay it aside, as an outworn garment. But in the meantime, we need to take care of it as a faithful servant who serves us well.

The body has an innate intelligence and it will outpicture that which we instruct it to do (either consciously or subconsciously), assisted by the body elemental, our guardian angel, and our Higher Self. Healthy thoughts and feelings are food for the body as well as the soul. If we love our body, it will respond to that love.

Our Higher Self sees us as perfect and whole, manifesting the original divine pattern, the perfect design for each of us and our life. Mothers in this world often have the gift of seeing their children in this light. They see the perfect, the beautiful, the lovable, even when their children are misbehaving or manifesting anything but these things. In the same way, it is the Divine Mother who holds this vision for each of our souls.

HEALTHY THOUGHTS AND FEELINGS ARE FOOD FOR THE
BODY AS WELL AS THE SOUL. IF WE LOVE OUR BODY, IT
WILL RESPOND TO THAT LOVE.

A friend gave me a wall plaque of the Blessed Virgin that she brought back from a trip to Colombia. I placed it near my bathroom mirror so that I could see it each day, even as I used a simple exercise to help me see myself as she sees me—in the image of the divine perfection of my Higher Self.

Each day as I stood before my mirror, I prayed and asked Mother Mary to purify all my past perceptions of my own imperfections. After this prayer, I would look into my own eyes in the mirror and practice seeing my eyes as Mary sees them. Our eyes have been described as "windows of the soul through which God can gaze joyfully upon all his creation." They tell the story of our past experiences. "Everything you have ever beheld tells its story as it was recorded in your eyes." Daily I practiced seeing myself and others as my Higher Self would see me. For what we see in others appears more readily in ourselves.[8]

The images that we hold in our mind's eye can work for or against us in healing. This is one reason why it is important to hold an image of perfection. This does not mean that we ignore what is happening to the physical body. We may know that we are fighting cancer, but we do not think of ourselves as ill. We must hold an image of good health in our mind's eye. Many mind-body techniques, such as the positive affirmations that Louise Hay teaches for healing, are tools to help us hold that image of perfection and make it more real to the conscious and subconscious minds. As this image is held steady in the mind, the body works to manifest it in the physical.

GEMSTONES AND CRYSTALS AS FOCUSES OF LIGHT

For many years I have owned and used crystals and gemstones, both as jewelry and as sources of light and healing. I have crystals at my personal altar in my home and at the altar that I keep in a small corner of my office, and I used them while dealing with cancer as tools to help heal my body of the cancer and the effects of the treatments.

The belief in the subtle spiritual influence of gemstones is ancient, and different gemstones have traditionally been associated with different qualities of spiritual energy. We find these traditions even in the Bible, where we read of the breastplate of the high priest containing twelve gemstones and John's vision of the New Jerusalem with twelve types of precious stones in its foundations.[9] The ancient knowledge of gems and crystals and the energies they can convey is being rediscovered today, and there are numerous comprehensive sources available on this subject.

Gemstones and crystals can store and transmit spiritual energy or light. Our spiritual centers (or chakras) are also storehouses for light and are intended to shine like jewels, but in most of us, these centers can only contain so much light. In times of challenge, and even facing the challenges of daily life, we can use the light of gemstones and crystals to give us additional assistance and increments of energy.

Certain gems and crystals are ideally suited to holding energy. These can be dedicated to this purpose, and when you wear them, they accumulate the energy of your prayers and devotions. The energy can then be released to you as you need it.

The energy of gems and crystals seems to work on higher levels—mental, emotional, and spiritual—and as with Bach Flower Remedies and similar healing tools, the effects may not be immediately apparent in the physical. However, as these subtle energies cycle through all the levels of being, they can be seen and felt manifesting in subtle but powerful ways.

Amethyst

Amethyst is an important gemstone for healing. It particularly amplifies the energies of the violet ray, the ray of change and transmutation.

The understanding of the spiritual properties of amethyst goes back a long way. The ancients believed the amethyst quelled any kind of passion, appetites, and desires of the body, that it helped control emotions, and that it imparted dignity, love, compassion, and hope. The Hebrews believed that it could induce dreams and visions.

Edgar Cayce said that the amethyst makes the body more sensitive to spiritual influences, higher vibrations, and healing forces. It's good to wear for meditation. Amethyst was one of the gemstones in the breastplate of the high priest and today is the gem in the bishop's ring in the Catholic and Episcopal Churches. It is associated with kingship, religious ceremony, and ritual in church and state. Amethyst is the gemstone of the alchemist and the prophet. It attracts the gifts of the Holy Spirit.[10]

I like to wear amethyst, and I always have an amethyst crystal on my desk—for resolution, harmony, joy, creativity, and freedom. I visualize the amethyst on my desk as a nexus in the exchange of energy between myself and those with whom I am meeting, whether on the phone or in person. I see a figure-eight flow of violet energy through all deliberations and conversations.

Jade

I was also drawn to other stones during my illness, some of which are known for their healing properties. I was particularly attracted to jade. In fact, three months before my diagnosis, while visiting friends in Russia, I became ill with flu-like symptoms and a sore throat. My Russian companion slipped a jade bracelet on my wrist and told me to wear it for healing, which I did. I remembered it when I was dealing with breast cancer and began to wear it again.

My mother sent me a beautiful jade pendant of Kuan Yin, known in the East as the goddess of mercy and compassion. The pendant came from China. It was two inches tall and one inch wide and delicately carved. I loved to wear my Kuan Yin pendant and found that it carried a healing and peaceful presence. I wore it over my heart for many months during my treatment. People often commented on it. It seemed to have an energy that they noticed. (I am wearing it in the picture on the cover of this book.)

I found out more about jade and its properties from *Love Is in the Earth: A Kaleidoscope of Crystals,* a reference book about gemstones with descriptions of the metaphysical properties of the mineral kingdom. I learned that jade is said to "inspire wisdom during the assessment of problems." It helps to "balance one's needs with the requirements of the day" and helps to care for that which is most important. It is known as a "dream stone"—it is used to "release suppressed emotions via the dream process."[11] (I certainly began to have dreams that aided me in my healing.)

Green jade is particularly known for its healing energy and as a focus of the emerald ray associated with healing. If I missed wearing my jade, I noticed it. It became a kind of talisman for me—but much more than a traditional lucky stone. I felt protected when wearing it, particularly during the difficult periods when I was choosing which course of treatment to take and during chemotherapy.

I thought of the phrase in the Bible, "And it shall come to pass, that before they call, I will answer."[12] Even before I knew that I needed it, I had received a piece of jade that helped me in my healing.

Ruby

Ruby is another gemstone that can be used for healing, but it needs some caution. It carries an energy that is not suitable for everyone and can stir the passions and aggravate anger or irritation in some people. Before my illness I could not wear it, as it had adverse effects on me. However, through an interesting incident I found that I was able to wear ruby easily after my treatment.

For years, my sister and I wore similar rings set with heart-shaped gemstones—mine an amethyst and hers an emerald. One day, during a particularly stressful period prior to my diagnosis, I looked down during a meeting at work and found that the amethyst was gone. I was going through a second job change and my team was being disbanded. The stone fell out while I was meeting with them to let them know that they would be losing their jobs.

The loss of the stone from my favorite ring shook me, and I had to struggle to regain my composure during the meeting. I looked high and low, but I could never find the stone, and the gaping hole where the amethyst had been seemed symbolic of how my heart was feeling at the time.

Some months later, as I was recovering from surgery, I was thinking that I would like the extra protection of a gemstone to wear and thought of replacing the stone in this ring. A friend went with me to a local jeweler to find one. I wanted a stone that would be appropriate for my experience of dealing with cancer. My friend had spoken about the spiritual meaning of the breast-cancer experience and suggested that a ruby might remind me of the heart, the spiritual center closest to the site of the cancer.

I had been considering a pinker stone rather than the rich red of a ruby, which seemed too strong for my personality and was not something I had been able to wear comfortably before this. However, as we looked at different stones, I somehow felt that a ruby would be appropriate. The jeweler helped me choose a deep-pink ruby, which symbolized for me the initiation of the heart that I was going through with the cancer experience.

When I later consulted the book on gemstones, I found out why I had been drawn to this stone. The book states that the ruby "stimulates the heart chakra and assists one in the selection and attainment of one's ultimate values. It further stimulates the loving, emotional side toward nurturing, bringing spiritual wisdom, health, knowledge, and wealth.... It is an excellent shielding stone, protecting on all levels.... The ruby encourages one to follow bliss. It is said to light the darkness of one's life." The ruby is used in the healing of many disorders and can be used to "decrease the length of time required for chemicals and toxins to exit the body." (How appropriate for chemotherapy.) The energy of the ruby can assist in making decisions and in "in changing one's world, promoting creativity and expansiveness in awareness and manifestation."[13]

Now that I am well, I find that ruby has a positive effect. I do not wear the jade as often now, as I find that it is too cooling. It seems that the cancer experience has changed my constitution.

Other Stones

As I was learning more about the healing properties of gemstones, I visited a local gemstone merchant. I had passed his store many times but had never gone in, and when I walked in that morning there were no other customers, just the owner and me. I told him that I was about to go through chemotherapy and radiation for breast cancer and asked if there were some stones or crystals that could assist me.

He looked me right in the eye, paused, and then told me that he understood. His wife had gone through breast cancer some years earlier and was now doing well. We started talking and I told him that I really did not like the idea of the chemotherapy but that I wanted to get through it. He smiled and said that he was a Vietnam veteran: he understood intense experiences. He did not like Vietnam, but he had gotten through it.

It was exactly what I needed to hear. He did not say a lot, but he helped me by sharing of his own experience. His example of courage and endurance was exactly what I needed at that time.

He mentioned some stones that might assist me during treatment:

- **Tiger iron**: a stone composed of tiger's eye, red jasper and hematite, which is used to increase the counts of the red and white blood cells during chemotherapy, or at least to cause them not to be lowered.
- **Obsidian**: American Indians consider obsidian to be a sacred healing stone, used to strengthen bones or heal broken bones. Obsidian absorbs and dispels negativity. It should not be worn on the body.
- **Picture jasper**: used to stimulate the immune system.

- **Red jasper:** a healing stone for those undergoing prolonged hospitalization and for reversing low energy states.
- **Carnelian:** a red or fire stone prized for its ability to produce a sense of life, aliveness, and energy, which forces out and destroys negative energy. For example, it is said to deal with the leftover residues of chemotherapy agents.
- **Rose quartz:** a pink stone which is calming, gentle and soothing. It symbolizes the opening of the heart and represents divine love rather than human sympathy.
- **Moonstone:** a green colored stone which helps to keep the treatment from affecting more of the body than it needs to.
- **Blue lace agate:** a light blue stone also used to keep the treatment from affecting more of the body than it needs to. It educates the spirit as to what the treatment is intended to do—for example, chemotherapy is for the selective destruction of the cancer cells.
- **Quartz crystal:** instills discipline, purity, peace, protection, joy, order, hope, and concentration and dispels negativity.

I purchased some small stones, and he told me to hold them in my hands during chemotherapy. I was also attracted to two beautiful fluorite crystals I found in a cabinet near the door—swirling purple/violet and green colors, perfect for the visualization of the violet flame and green healing light. I left the store enriched by the experience in more ways than one.

The stones I have mentioned above are the ones towards which my Higher Self guided me. You may choose entirely different stones, depending on your circumstances and preferences. Chinese medicine teaches about five elements, with each person's constitution being composed of these elements in varying degrees. Depending on the ratios of these elements, different gemstones may have different effects on different people. Your choice of gemstones will be guided by your constitution and also the specific energy that you need. For example, jade is known for its cooling effect. Chemotherapy and radiation are of the fire element, and jade can help cool the fire.

If you are interested in adding gemstones or crystals to your program of healing, a good place to start would be to get a book or find information online about their spiritual properties. See what resonates for you and meets your needs. You could also go to a gemstone and crystal shop and hold different stones in your hand to feel their unique energy. However, if you are looking for somewhere to begin, you can't go wrong with amethyst.

A HOUSE CALLED HOPE

Across the street from the hospital where I received my treatment were three houses where out-of-town patients could stay while undergoing outpatient treatment. I stayed in one of these houses for six weeks of radiation.

The hospital staff named these houses "Faith," "Hope," and "Charity." I lived in the middle house, "Hope." This was very appropriate, because I had been thinking a lot about hope.

I became aware of the power of hope in the days after my first biopsy, when I knew that I had breast cancer but did not know how serious it was. I had not yet had a lymph-node biopsy, and I wondered if the cancer had spread to my lymph nodes or perhaps even to my bones or lungs. A chest X-ray had not shown any obvious metastases, and I had no symptoms—but then, I had had no symptoms from the breast lump either.

My emotions were on the "roller coaster" that everyone talks about. At times, I was in the depths of despair, feeling that I might have only a few months or years to live. At other times, I felt that I was going to fight this thing with my last breath and be victorious. And sometimes I thought that, given the facts, it could well be stage I (i.e., no sign of the cancer having spread to the lymph nodes) and the outcome would probably be good.

I was having trouble sleeping. I would wake up at 3 A.M. and wake Peter up, asking him to hug me and talk to me. I couldn't eat properly and walked about in a daze.

I received my first real infusion of hope from a seemingly unexpected source. It was during the first appointment I had with the oncologist I saw in Montana. I have already related how he looked at me at the very end of the interview and said, "You know you are not going to die. Your outlook is probably very good." This had a very big impact. I had not realized that midst the ups and downs I was carrying an overlay of depression. Suddenly, after feeling so down, I felt a *whole* lot better. My spirits soared. I practically danced out of the hospital. "Why, he thinks I am going to live!"

Six months later, here I was, living in a house called Hope. It seemed that the angels were really trying to get me to think about this. I came to realize that hope is an essential ingredient in the healing process. Hope even affects the functioning of the immune system—in those who don't have any hope of recovery, the immune system stops working well and their own thoughts become a self-fulfilling prophecy.

Although my cancer was not as serious as many and my outcome was likely to be good, I found that holding on to hope was still a challenge. There is such a weight that comes from the diagnosis—everything that you read and all the people that you know who have died from it. Even being in a hospital with other cancer patients can be like a two-edged sword. You can get the best treatment there, but seeing other cancer patients, especially those with more serious cases, reminds you of your own illness. All of this can hang over you like a dark cloud.

Hope is the golden ray of the sun piercing that cloud. It is a grace, but it is also something that we can win and attain. Hope can come from many sources, including prayer, mental determination, and even grace.

At the same time, you do not want to be either too optimistic or like an ostrich burying your head in the sand, not paying attention to the seriousness of your condition. For here in your body is something that will eventually take your life—if it is allowed to continue. You need to be very realistic in order to make good choices. And as you seek to balance hope and realism, it sometimes feels as though you are walking a tightrope.

I believe that for hope to be effective, it must be anchored in reality. Just "hoping" that the cancer will go away by itself is not hope but a retreat into fantasy. Hope is the rope that you pull on to get you through the hard times—the painful physical, mental, and emotional changes you deal with in cancer. Change is always painful, since you have to let go of something familiar, even loved, before you can accept something new.

I believe that there is always room for hope, no matter what the diagnosis or the statistics. Even if the statistics are 99 percent against us, there is nothing that says that we cannot be the one in a hundred who makes it. No one is a statistic. Everyone is an individual.

Bernie Siegel says he would much rather know about the individual patient than about the statistics—what the patient brings to the challenge is a much more reliable guide to the likely outcome. He also points out that hope is always an option:

> If nine out of ten people with a certain disease are expected to die of it, supposedly you are spreading "false hope" unless you tell *all ten* they'll probably die. Instead, I say each person could be the one who survives, because all hope is real in the patient's mind....
>
> Even if what you most hope for—a complete cure—doesn't come to pass, the hope itself can sustain you to accomplish many things in the meantime. Refusal to hope is nothing more than a decision to die. I know there are many people alive today because I gave them hope and told them they didn't have to die.[14]

I also believe that hope is always an option because healing is always an option. In the highest sense, hope is not about living or dying but how we face the day. No matter what the physical outcome, healing is always possible for the heart and the soul. We will all leave our bodies behind one day, and it is the heart and the soul that we take with us, even after the physical body is gone.

CHECKLIST: SPIRITUALITY AND HEALING

✓ **Scientific studies show that prayer works.** Start to harness the power of prayer for healing.

✓ **Talk to God, commune with him, and listen for his answers.**

✓ **Pray scientifically and combine prayer with focused visualizations.**

✓ **Be specific in your prayers.** For example pray that the chemotherapy only go where it is intended to go in your body, that it not damage any healthy cells, that white-cell counts and blood counts are not be reduced too much, and that there are not unwanted side effects.

✓ **Enlist the help of other "prayer warriors"** by asking them to pray for and with you. Share your specific prayers with them.

✓ **Let your prayer partners know how you are doing.** Regular progress reports help them to know what to pray for.

✓ **Harness the power of the spoken Word in your prayers.**

✓ **Hold the image of perfection for yourself,** and ask others to also see you in this way.

✓ **Use meditation to boost your immune system, increase awareness and overcome side effects.** Find a method that appeals to you and fits with your beliefs.

✓ **Use gemstones and crystals to focus light and healing energy.** You can't go wrong with an amethyst.

✓ **Hold on to hope.** Even if the odds are not good, there is nothing to say you won't be the one who makes it.

CHAPTER 15

GETTING THROUGH CHEMO

I consider getting through chemotherapy the biggest challenge on my journey through cancer, and in a way, my biggest achievement. I was so grateful to be finally through it.

Every patient's experience with chemotherapy is different. There are different drugs and different dosages, depending on the type of cancer, and different drugs have different side effects.

There are a few people who appear to sail through chemotherapy with very little trouble, but they are definitely the minority. Most experience side effects and encounter significant challenges, and a few have serious complications.

Overall, I think I did well. I fought hard and did the very best that I could. I tried to create the most favorable environment for myself to get through it. I can't point to any single thing as the key ingredient (except perhaps a determination to endure). I found that it was putting all these things together that was the recipe for me to have a good outcome.

In this chapter I share the things that helped me. They may help you or a loved one or give you clues to finding your own path for "getting through chemo."

SIDE EFFECTS

There is no question that chemotherapy is intense. It was a frightening sensation to feel those chemicals going into my body, knowing the potential side effects. I almost felt that I had to be alert and vigilant so that the good cells would not be harmed.

Many of the side effects of chemotherapy—such as nausea and hair loss—are well-known, and I was expecting them. However, chemotherapy affects almost every system in the body in some way, and there are many other effects, great and small. Talk to your doctor, do your research, and find out what to expect in the way of side effects for your particular prescription. This will give you the best chance to be prepared to deal with them if they do arise.

"CHEMO-BRAIN"

One effect I was not expecting was that chemotherapy made me forgetful and fuzzy in my thinking at times. Patients and doctors call it "chemo-brain"—it's like your head is full of cotton wool. It is hard to study or concentrate on anything except television or light reading.

In planning for my first chemotherapy treatment, I could see myself sitting in a comfortable chair at the hospital for a week with nothing to do but catch up on my reading. I took all kinds of books, only to find that I simply could not get into them. The nurses told me that many chemo patients do this—they come in armed with books to study, only to find that chemo-brain takes over. Another effect of chemo-brain is that it makes it hard to have a sense of control over your life and circumstances, since you become absent-minded and have difficulty focusing on tasks.

Spiritually and energetically, I could feel the chemo entering and leaving my body. I would breathe a sigh of relief when, a few days after the end of the chemo session, it was finally eliminated from my body. It felt as if an unwelcome houseguest had gone and I could finally be alone in my own body.

NAUSEA

Nausea and tiredness are the twin companions of most cancer patients. For me, the nausea and the sick feeling while the chemotherapy was going in and for a few days afterwards was the most difficult part of the experience. It is hard to describe how bad constant nausea makes you feel. There is nowhere to go and nowhere to hide to get away from it.

I tried a number of different things for the nausea, but I never found the magic bullet. The doctors prescribed antinausea medication, which seemed to help somewhat. They also suggested Sea-Bands, elastic cuffs that are worn over acupressure points on the wrists. I took several herbal and homeopathic medicines. Getting up and walking helped, as did gentle exercise and stretching. All these things seemed to work together to keep the nausea at a manageable level. However, it was still bad enough that a couple of days into each treatment I did not feel like eating much, if at all.

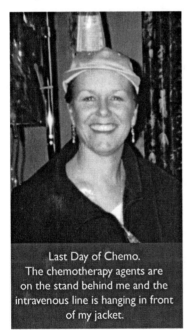

Last Day of Chemo. The chemotherapy agents are on the stand behind me and the intravenous line is hanging in front of my jacket.

There seems to be a strong mind-body component to nausea, as I found out from one very interesting experience. On the evening of my last day of chemotherapy, Peter talked me into going with him to see the new *Star Wars* movie that had just been released. Because of my nausea, I didn't feel much like going, but he was looking forward to it, and I thought it might take my mind off things. Besides, if I was going to be feeling bad it would not make much difference if I was sitting in a movie theater or a hotel room.

As it turned out, I became absorbed in the movie, and when we walked out I was amazed to realize that for those two hours I had not felt tired or nauseated at all. Once the movie was over the nausea soon returned, and I did not seem to be able to get back to that place where the movie had taken me, where I was no longer aware of feeling sick. However, I certainly learned something about the power of the mind.

TIREDNESS

After the shock of the initial diagnosis and the subsequent surgery, I was tired and drained. They say that sleep deprivation is cumulative. I felt that I could have slept for months and still not been replenished. Initially, I spent a number of days in bed just resting and recovering. This soon stretched into several weeks of sleeping in and lounging around in my nightgown. Once I felt that I had gotten the rest I needed, I decided to get up and get dressed each morning after Peter went to work.

By the time the chemotherapy treatments started, I was as ready as I could be. I made sure that I got all the sleep that I needed, but I also got up each day because I had work to do. I was a cancer-fighter. I decided that I would think of fighting cancer as a job. That included taking good care of myself.

Tiredness is one of the things that you expect with chemotherapy, but I was generally very fortunate with this—it only really affected me during the treatment. When I was tired, I took time to get the rest I needed and to adjust my activity to my energy level, and I found I would be fine after a few days. I think the exercise and other therapies I used helped raise my energy level in general so that the usual tiredness that goes with chemotherapy did not affect me as much as it does many people.

LOOK GOOD, FEEL BETTER

When you are feeling ill, you would think that the last thing you would care about is your appearance. In one sense this is true, and there are some people who are blessed to be completely unconcerned about their appearance at any time.

However, I also know firsthand that looking in the mirror can be quite depressing on days when you feel and look unwell. Depression is something you don't need when you are trying to boost your immune system. Furthermore, how you look and feel also affects how others treat you.

I had seen many cancer patients in my years as a medical doctor, and I did not want to see myself become or even look like a "cancer patient." On my hospital visits, I noted the patients who looked good. In some ways their appearance seemed to suggest that they were on top of their situation, and I looked to them for inspiration. (I do not mean to denigrate anyone's appearance. I know that there are times when we cannot look good and the effects of our illness show through. But I know that doing my best to look good was helpful for me and for my own healing.) For me, an important part of looking good was the clothes I wore.

Former cancer patients told me that after treatment you will never want to wear your "chemo clothes" again because they will remind you of the treatment sessions. They were right. I heard of patients making a celebratory bonfire of their chemo clothes after their treatment. I decided to buy specific clothes for chemotherapy, which I could throw away once I was done.

In the midst of treatment, when you may feel tired and nauseous, comfortable clothes can make a big difference. And due to all the tests and examinations, you will find that you have to get in and out of your outfits frequently. Many patients are very happy wearing tracksuits or jeans, and I sometimes wore these too. However, I also tried to find outfits that had some style. For me, this was not a time for drab and dingy colors. I purchased some inexpensive but attractive clothes that suited me, were easy to get on and off, and were comfortable to lounge around in. I was glad I did.

When not in chemo, I took care to look good and dress well, even if it was just for me. I found out that if I made the effort to look good, it really did help me to feel better. It boosted my spirits—and probably my immune system as well. It always gave me a lift when people told me that I looked great. I think they were happy to see that I didn't look like a cancer "victim" or what they imagined a cancer patient would look like. I looked and felt like someone who was going to live.

NURTURING MYSELF

For several months before my diagnosis, I had felt the need to nurture and take care of myself in a better way. I had returned to the local hot springs after not having gone there for some time, and I had started to work on getting more exercise.

After the diagnosis and after I had done everything I needed to for my treatment, I then made taking care of myself a priority. I felt a great need to nurture myself, and I developed a routine of self-care. I took time showering, using a soft bristle brush and later a cactus-fiber cloth. I applied lotions and essential oils to my body and my hair. I took time to cleanse, tone, and moisturize my face. I played uplifting music or mantras. I wore makeup—even when I was unlikely to see anyone. I painted my nails (something that I had not done in years).

Many cancer centers teach that addressing the physical changes that come with cancer and its treatment is an important part of the healing process. This can lead to a more positive attitude, greater self-esteem, increased personal comfort, and a greater sense of well-being. This was very true for me.

My mother and sister were very generous and sent me "glad money" with which to pamper myself. They knew me very well and wanted to cheer me up even though they could not be physically present with me. When you are not earning an income and money is tight because of medical bills, gifts from friends and family can be a real blessing. Thanks to my family, I was able to consult a beautician and makeup expert to get a makeover and to seek advice on natural skin-care products. I also treated myself to a visit to a day spa and had a facial, manicure, and body massage. These visits always boosted my spirits, helped me relax, and took my mind off the cancer and the treatment. They also helped to give me a sense of control over my life.

An interesting incident illustrated this principle for me. A friend had sent me a small sample bottle of a very expensive moisturizing product. I used it and really liked the effect that it had on my face. When it ran out, I could not find it anywhere in Montana. A girlfriend from Minneapolis called and asked if there was anything at all that she could do. Would I like anything?

I sheepishly told her about the product that I could not find. It seemed so silly even to mention it, given everything else that was going on in my life. But she, bless her heart, took the time to track down a bottle at Bloomingdales and send it to me. It was like getting a Christmas package in April. It made me feel very special, and that bottle of lotion did a tremendous amount to boost my morale. Looking back, I think that this incident sent a message to my body that I loved it and was willing to spend time and energy to nurture it. Bernie Siegel calls this sending a "live" message.

As I began to take good care of my body, the results were evident. My skin looked better and more radiant than I could ever remember, although I am sure that better diet, vitamins, and exercise (not to mention prayer) also helped. I lost the weight I had gained in the previous few years and had more energy than I had had in some time.

People came up to me to tell me that I looked really well. When I looked in the mirror, I could tell that I was looking better than I had in years. I even looked younger.

SKIN CARE AND COSMETICS

Skin care can be very important for those undergoing chemotherapy and radiation treatment. Chemotherapy patients often find that they develop dry skin and need moisturizers. Certain types of cytotoxic drugs can also produce photosensitivity (abnormal sensitivity of the skin to light), and that means staying out of the sun and using a good sunscreen.

One tip we received in image-enhancement classes at the hospital was to avoid the possibility of bacterial infections from mascara or other cosmetics that are used for long periods of time. Mascara should be replaced every few months, and products should be taken from their containers via spatulas or cotton buds so that the container is not contaminated with bacteria that might be picked up from the skin. Usually these small traces of bacteria would not be a problem, but when the immune system is weakened by chemotherapy, even small things can become much more significant.

I found that more natural products, preferably organic, were definitely better for my body. They were a little more expensive, but they were worth the extra cost for the way that they made me feel. Also, unnecessary chemicals can be an added load on your immune system. When you think about it, you can absorb a lot of lipstick and makeup into your body during a lifetime.

Some of the other skincare products that I used included vitamin-E cream for the breasts to help reduce scarring from surgery and to help the skin deal with the effects of radiation, Melaleuca (Australian tea tree oil) and arnica ointment to help with the disinfection and healing of intravenous sites, comfrey and golden seal cream, and chamomile cream.

SPECIAL NEEDS FOR SPECIAL PEOPLE

Chemotherapy and radiation are administered to kill cancer cells, which divide and grow rapidly. However, they also affect any other cells in the body that divide quickly, such as those in the hair follicles, the skin, and the mucous membranes of the mouth and the gastrointestinal system. The death of these rapidly-dividing cells usually causes the hair to fall out at the root and can produce mouth ulcers and other problems with the digestive system. Fortunately, I did not suffer from mouth ulcers or intestinal problems. However, I did lose some hair.

Hair loss usually occurs two to three weeks after the first chemotherapy session. The rate of hair loss depends on the individual.

Several days before the hair loss or during it, you may feel pain, itchiness, or sensitivity in your scalp. All body hair may be affected during chemotherapy, but scalp hair is faster growing than most other body hair and therefore often affected more. Hair loss may range from thinning to complete baldness. The hair usually does not grow back until three to six weeks after chemotherapy has ended.

My fellow patients have told me that hair loss was one of the most difficult things to cope with during chemotherapy—even though it is less important medically because it is hardly life-threatening. Many felt embarrassed about hair loss. Some felt a little guilty about being concerned about it, because they had more "important" things to worry about. But hair loss is often the most visible sign that something is wrong and that you are indeed a cancer patient. Walking down the street, no one knows that you are undergoing cancer treatment until you lose your hair. It makes you stand out and feel self-conscious.

Cancer Treatment Centers of America has a Cosmetic Image Enhancement program to provide support, information, and resources for cancer patients on how to look good during treatment. One two-hour session I attended was given by Lori Irsay, owner of Salon 475 and creator of a program called Special Needs for Special People.

Lori has a great sense of humor and a knack for putting people at ease. Her presentations on image enhancement covered everything from how to deal with hair loss (including wigs, fashion turbans, hats, and head covers) to makeup tips. Lori teaches patients how to make the most of their facial features while undergoing hair loss, which may include loss of eyebrows and eyelashes.

Often the first thought people have about hair loss is to get a wig. However, some people I know bought wigs and rarely wore them. They were too hot and uncomfortable, and perhaps most importantly, they would say, "It's just not me." But if you are having chemotherapy for a year, then it may well be worth the investment, especially for important occasions.

Lori teaches that there are wigs and there are wigs—from the very cheap synthetic wigs to the expensive $2,000 human-hair wigs. There is a difference, and you do not have to go top of the line to get something that works well. With Lori's help, I tried on several in the $200 to $500 range that looked really good on me and quite natural. It put me at ease to know that if I ever needed to wear a wig I would feel comfortable doing so.

It is important to be properly fitted for a wig by a specialist. Lori showed me wigs where the hair is attached to a mesh crown that looks like a normal scalp. Wigs can be cut and styled to suit you. There are also several mail-order wig catalogs available, although it might be hard to get a good fit from a catalog.

If you get a prescription from your doctor for a wig, your insurance plan may cover some or all of the cost. (Your doctor might prescribe "Cranial hair prosthesis for medical purposes. Alopecia secondary to chemotherapy or radiation therapy.")

I learned a lot about looking good from Lori and thoroughly enjoyed the experience. There are probably people near you that can help with such information and services. Take advantage of them. My local cosmetologist and hair stylist in Montana became so interested in learning how to help me that she attended a half-day training session on dealing with the cosmetic side of cancer treatment. She is now able to help others who come to her.

HAIR—WHO NEEDS IT?

My oncologist had told me that I would most likely lose my hair, and I thought that I was prepared for it. Nevertheless, it took me by surprise when it happened. I was paying attention to other matters and working hard at avoiding other side effects when I began to notice little hairs everywhere. After two days of seeing hairs on my pillow, it still did not register that this was due to the chemotherapy. It finally hit me one day when I saw how much hair was collecting at the bottom of the shower. Then I noticed that quite a bit of hair would come out every time I ran my fingers over my head. Hairs were everywhere—on the sofa, in the bed, on the floor, on my shoulders. For a while I stopped wearing dark colors.

From that point, I spent a lot of time wondering about what to do if the hair loss got worse. Wear a hat? Shave it off and go beautifully bald? Wear scarves or turbans? Wear a wig?

I was pretty much prepared to go bald if I needed to. A friend had been standing at a beauty counter next to a very fashionable bald woman who was beautifully made up, and she returned to tell me that she could not wait to see me bald, as she thought I would look really good.

I tried a number of things to give myself the best chance to keep some hair. I had read that satin pillowcases were helpful in preventing hair loss. They are intended to reduce friction on the hair and therefore cause less discomfort and less hair loss. I am not sure if they did, but they certainly felt very smooth and nice against my skin.

I saw a hairstylist early in my treatment and three weeks prior to chemotherapy she recommended some hair-care products by Nioxin specifically formulated to prevent hair loss. I used these products during my treatment and as I recovered, and I believe that they were part of what helped me retain some of my hair. They are relatively expensive, but I treated myself with the funds that my mother and sister sent me.

I also used some herbal products on my hair during the chemotherapy phase. I rinsed my hair with stinging nettle tea. I also made up a special formula of oil, which I applied to my hair each day. It consisted of burdock oil, Saint John's wort oil, and borage oil in a base of olive oil. I made the burdock oil by simmering burdock roots in olive oil. I added the Saint John's wort oil from a bottled source, and the borage oil I squeezed out of capsules. I poured all of this into a bottle and applied the mixture to my hair each day. Before my shower I would apply the oil to my head and leave it to soak for an hour. I would then shampoo with the Nioxin products. My hair looked healthy and shiny and felt very soft.

On my second visit, the oncologist seemed surprised that I had so much hair left and told me that maybe I would not lose all my hair after all. As it turned out, my hair thinned all over, and then it worsened in certain areas, particularly the front of the hairline and the top of the crown. Peter joked about male-pattern baldness. I began to brush my hair back off my face to cover the bald spots. I eventually lost half to two thirds of my hair. My scalp ached a little for a few days around the time when it really started falling out. I also lost some eyelashes and half my body hair, including my pubic hair.

I wore scarves, baseball caps, and a variety of hats when it was thinnest. Prior to that, when I first noticed it falling out, I had had it cut short in anticipation of further hair loss. I was very glad that I did, as it made the hair loss seem less noticeable. The hairs were shorter and less distressing to see. There was less of a mess, and it generally felt better. After a while, I got used to hair loss, and it did not bother me as much.

Whether you lose your hair or not, there are ways to cope. Scarves can look really good and can complement an outfit. If I wasn't sure if I wanted to wear one, I would wear it around my neck and be ready to tie it on my head. Livingston, Montana, is known as one of the windiest cities in the United States, and a scarf was often useful.

Claudia, a fellow patient, had lost most of her hair following her first chemotherapy session and had shaved off the rest. She looked stunning in a baseball cap over her bald head. We shared a room for chemotherapy, and inspired by her, I sought to develop my own style.

After Claudia introduced me to baseball caps, I found several on sale at Wal-Mart. White and khaki went with many of my outfits. They were jaunty and made me feel sporty—they helped me remember I was in cancer-fighting mode. I also bought a Greek fisherman's cap on sale, which I really enjoyed wearing.

One night, just for fun, Peter and I had a fashion parade of different hats. Peter ended up taking some photos, and the results are shown in this chapter. We laughed at all the different looks and sent photos to our families: the "Jackie O" look, with the scarf tied under the chin and dark glasses; the "Maggie Tabberer" look, named after a famous Australian fashion model who wore stunningly short hair pulled back off her face; and "Neroli of the North," wearing a sheepskin hat with ear flaps. (You might get away with this in Montana in the winter.) Peter liked me best in baseball caps and the fisherman's hat. We had fun looking at hair loss as an opportunity to make a fashion statement rather than something simply to be endured.

During and after chemotherapy, when my hair was very short and thin, on several occasions men came up to me while shopping to say that they really liked my hair and wished that their wives would adopt a similar style. It often provoked an interesting conversation when I explained that the hairstyle was courtesy of chemotherapy!

LESSONS FROM LOSING MY HAIR

In the midst of losing half my hair, I recalled something that I had said from the time I was first married. Pete is one of those guys who doesn't really notice what you are wearing. It used to annoy me at first, but I soon came to see that it did not matter to him how I looked, he simply loved me for who I was. I told myself that I could be old and wrinkled one day, and he would still see me as young and lovely. I began to see that as a blessing.

Before getting cancer I had even joked with my hairdresser that Peter would never notice a change in hairstyle or even hair color. We would laugh, and after each style change, she would ask me if he noticed. He usually didn't unless I gave him advance warning. In fact, I used to joke that I could turn up bald and he would still not notice. Well, here I was, nearly bald, and he, of course, did notice, but loved me just the same.

I also learned something about the mind-body connection. I was already aware of the fascinating fact that in chemotherapy trials, patients who received placebos could actually lose their hair if told that it was a side effect of the product they were using.[1] The body seemed to obey what the mind was telling it to do, a theory I was able to confirm in my own experience with hair loss.

Since hair loss due to chemotherapy is only temporary and not life threatening, initially I was much more worried about other side effects.

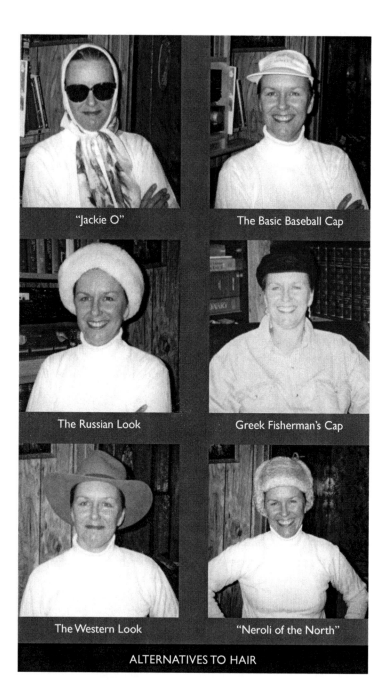

"Jackie O"

The Basic Baseball Cap

The Russian Look

Greek Fisherman's Cap

The Western Look

"Neroli of the North"

ALTERNATIVES TO HAIR

During one of my talks with my body elemental and my Higher Self, I told my body that it was to avoid side effects during chemotherapy, but if it had to manifest a side effect, then I would not mind hair loss. It would be better than low white-cell counts or diarrhea or weight loss.

Well, my body took me at my word. I had given it permission to lose my hair, and that is what it did. I hoped for the best and prepared for the worst, and in my earnest desire to be prepared for all eventualities, I even began to visualize myself bald to prepare myself for this eventuality.

After I had lost about half of my hair, I realized that I had actually been sending a message to my body that the hair should go. At this point I was getting very little in the way of other side effects, and my body was coping very well. Was it really necessary to lose my hair?

I decided to send a different message. I spoke to my body elemental and Higher Self each night before bed and gave specific instructions. I told my body to stop losing hair, and within three days, it did. I had very little additional hair loss from that time on. If I ever needed to know the power of thought to influence my body, here was the proof.

My advice to someone about to undergo chemotherapy and who is worried about potential hair loss is the following: Have a serious talk to your body. Explain that you do not want to lose your hair and that it is to hold onto that hair very firmly by the roots. Visualize your hair as full and healthy. Take care of it with good products.

If it happens that you do not lose your hair, then glory to God and praise to your body elemental! If you do lose your hair, it is not the end of the world. Take it in your stride, seek to look and feel good anyway, and make the best of the situation with all of the help at your disposal. Be creative. Find your own style. Think about famous people who are bald and beautiful, like Michael Jordan, Bernie Siegel, and Demi Moore in *G.I. Jane*.

There is also a spiritual perspective to losing your hair. The hair on your head grows at a rate of about half an inch per month, so six inches of hair is like a timeline of the last year of your life. Spiritually speaking, your hair carries the records of your life, the burdens and stresses you have carried in recent months and years. Losing your hair can be symbolic of new beginnings—losing the old self and putting on the new. Peter pointed out one day that if you were entering a Buddhist monastery, your head would be shaved as a sign of initiation and the leaving behind of your old life.

Everyone is different as to how they feel about losing their hair. Some of my fellow patients wore their baldness proudly and looked great. Others looked great in a baseball cap, a stylish turban, or a hat. I had several friends who looked very smart in their wigs. Loss of one's hair is a humbling experience, and in the end I kind of enjoyed even that too. If I were to have chemotherapy again and lose some of my hair, I might shave it all off and start again.

Hair loss is simply another reminder that you never know what to expect in life and you cannot always control it. However, you can make the best of whatever life throws your way.

SPIRITUAL TECHNIQUES

During chemotherapy, I used a number of spiritual techniques, which I have spoken about in previous chapters. I had my gemstones and crystals, used visualization and imagery, and used music and laughter. During this time, I especially learned about the power of prayer and mantra.

I said a prayer over the plastic bags containing the chemotherapy agents before they went into my body. I blessed them by placing my hands on them and asking that they be charged with light. I often placed a picture of a favorite saint over the bag, attached by a rubber band. I visualized the chemotherapy as liquid light entering my body. I saw it as brilliant violet/blue/green light, the colors of transformation, protection, and healing.

I prayed that the chemotherapy agents would go only to the cancer or to wherever they were needed in my body. I specifically asked that the chemotherapy not harm healthy cells and tissues. (I gave the same instruction to my body during the radiation treatment, and I saw the radiation as the X-rays of God going into my body and filling it with light.)

Prayer often sustained me when I was feeling the effects of the medication, yet at those times it felt as if my faith were being tested, because the medication made it hard to feel the effects of prayer. At times I felt as if I were encased in lead. The subtle vibrations of spiritual energy or the sense of contact with God I could normally feel when I prayed or meditated or gave mantras seemed to be much diminished in the midst of chemotherapy. I remember feeling that my prayers were not going very far, almost as if they would go two inches above my head and then fizzle out. I would often feel numb and somewhat cut off from the light. Other patients told me that they also found it harder to pray or had a sense that their prayers were somehow less effective.

These are the tests that come with cancer that people rarely speak about. Cancer is not just a physical trial—as inconvenient and painful as it might be physically. It is also a spiritual test, often a "dark night" when everything seems bleak and lonely and God seems very far away.

After the second chemotherapy session I somehow concluded that my prayers were not really working, because I could not feel the light as I usually did. It was a real effort to focus on prayer and spiritual work in the midst of nausea and chemo-brain—especially when the spiritual work did not seem to be helping. So, on the third visit, I prayed less and relied more on the prayers of others.

I learned a very important lesson. There are times when we need to rely solely on the prayers of others. However, if we are still able to pray, then we should do our part. As a minister, I had often told people that prayer works whether you feel it working or not. Anyone who really knows prayer will tell you that the times you feel alone and cut off are exactly when you should keep praying. However, it can be hard to remember these things when you are suffering through a trial such as cancer.

I soon learned what a mistake it was to cut back on my own prayers. The third session was one of the more difficult of the four. I took it as a lesson, and I learned to let God be the judge of whether my prayers were working or not. What vanity to think that if I could not feel them, God could not answer.

During the fourth and final chemotherapy session, I prayed in a more centered and detached way. I visualized the prayers as pencil beams of light going up out of the earth's atmosphere to contact God and the angels. I found that this session went far better than the third one, and I also realized that I had just done my own clinical trial on the effectiveness of prayer.

Journal Entry
February 13, 1999
Meditation and thoughts on preparing for chemotherapy

I consciously let go and surrender my body, my breast, and the cancer to the care of the angels and to Mother Mary. I do not need to sacrifice myself or my body or any part of my body unless God wills it. I do not need to martyr myself. I am learning how to live rather than how to die. I breathe in peace and exhale tension. I breathe in love and exhale pain and grief.

My immune system is strong and healthy. Its mission is to clear the unhealthy cancer cells. My immune system recognizes unhealthy cells and eliminates them from my body. I send love throughout my body and dissolve the unhealthy cells. The cancer is becoming obvious to the immune cells and millions of healthy cells come to the rescue. The healthy immune cells seek out and recognize the unhealthy cells and remove them.

I have no fear of the cancer. I have no fear of the chemotherapy and the radiation. As the Bible says, I can eat any deadly thing and it will not hurt me. My body easily receives the chemotherapy and accepts the needles and the intravenous canulas. I feel calm and relaxed and there are no side effects. I feel good before, during, and after my treatments.

I am surrounded by love, prayers, and well wishes from those who love me. I am eating well, I have energy, and I do activities that I want to do. I am at peace. I am vibrant and calm. I am spiritually aware. I am satisfied with all that I am doing and becoming.

I feel strong, energetic, calm, and good. My mind is clear of all negativity. I am able to think well, to concentrate and focus. My heart, soul, mind, and body are healing, strengthening, and overcoming the cancer. I am relaxed and happy.

I am flooded with gratitude for God and his wondrous creation of me, my body, and my immune system. The all-seeing eye of God will help to find and eliminate the cancer cells. Together we eliminate that which I have created that is not of God and replace it with God-like qualities and virtues. All is well.

CHECKLIST: GETTING THROUGH CHEMO

✓ **Use medications to reduce side effects.** They are improving all the time—get recommendations from your oncologist.

✓ **Ask your medical staff for their recommendations.** They have pages of information and tips on diet and other techniques to help you get through chemo.

✓ **Try acupuncture to counteract nausea and other side effects.**

✓ **Mild or moderate exercise** helps boost your immune system, relax your body and change your perspective. Walk or do yoga, deep breathing, tai chi, gentle stretching—whatever feels comfortable.

✓ **Don't expect to be able to study or do intense mental work while the chemo is going in.**

✓ **Listen to your body.** Rest and sleep when you are tired.

✓ **Take care of yourself and allow others to help you.**

✓ **Try to look your best even if you don't feel your best.** "Look good, feel better" works for many people.

✓ **Have a set of comfortable and soft "chemo clothes" that you wear to treatment sessions.**

✓ **Bless your chemo.** Place your hands over it asking it to be charged with healing light.

✓ **Talk to your body.** Tell it what is happening and what you would like it to do.

✓ **Use spiritual healing methods.** Give chants or mantras. Pray and ask others to pray for you. Even if it feels like your prayers are not going anywhere, have faith that they are making a difference.

SECTION III

Cancer as Teacher

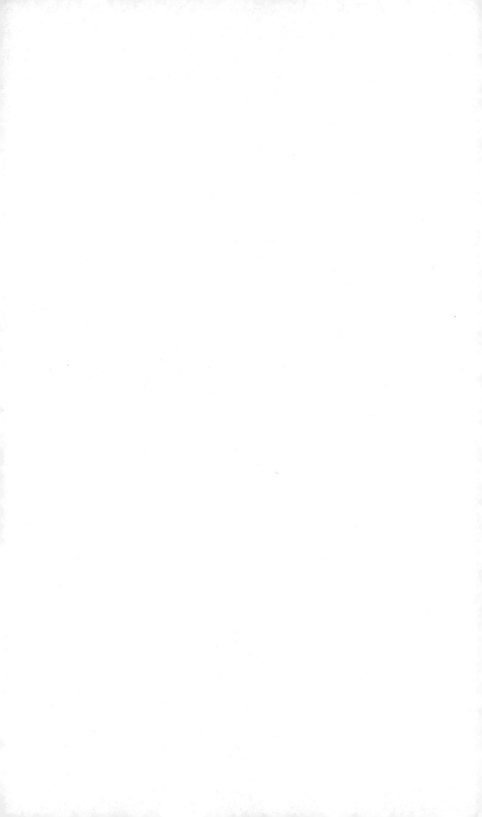

CHAPTER 16

ILLNESS AS A SPIRITUAL INITIATION

S o far in this book, you have read what I have learned and experienced as a doctor who became a breast-cancer patient. I have talked about treatments and what I did to find healing on all levels—physical, emotional, mental, and spiritual. What I am about to share is what I have learned about cancer from the perspective of the spiritual life and the evolution of the soul.

Some of these things I have learned from others. Some I have learned in the crucible of the cancer experience, and I can only say that they are true for me. They may not necessarily be true for others, although when I have shared these thoughts with other cancer patients, some have said that my experience mirrored their own. I hope that in speaking my truth, I will not offend others or their beliefs, for truly I respect all beliefs.

I believe that illness can be a teacher, presenting lessons that we may not be able to learn in any other way. I chose to see the experience of cancer in this light. Cancer certainly was a teacher to me—a hard one, seemingly even cruel at times, bringing me face to face with myself. Its messages were often unexpected. I had to be willing to listen, even if what I learned would be painful—and it certainly was painful at times.

Spiritually speaking, we can see cancer as a time of soul testing and spiritual initiation. I have not found any books on the subject of cancer as an initiation on the spiritual path. I can only share my experience and tell you what I gleaned from it.

ILLNESS CAN BE A TEACHER, PRESENTING LESSONS THAT WE MAY NOT BE ABLE TO LEARN IN ANY OTHER WAY.

TESTS IN LIFE

An Eastern adept once said that we will be tested in life as we walk the spiritual path, and that these tests are for the proving and perfecting of the soul. In fact, we do not choose the tests in life—they choose us.[1]

I think that this is true. I would never have chosen cancer as a means of initiation, but as I look back on the experience, I can see that it was all in divine order and that there was a higher purpose for it all. I learned so much and I gained so much. I cannot do anything but continue to praise God, for with every test, God also provides the means to pass that test.

I am often struck by the word "patient." It seems to imply waiting and having patience. Like all cancer patients, I often had to "hurry up and wait"—wait for the test results, wait for the doctor, wait for the chemotherapy to be finished, wait for the healing to take place. And perhaps this is as it should be.

Cancer does not appear overnight—this cancer had been growing in my breast for some time. The healing of cancer does not happen overnight, either. Like all healing, it takes patience. And yet, the diagnosis of cancer came upon me suddenly, and with it, the spiritual initiation of cancer began suddenly too—ready or not. It's like losing your hair—within a few days it can all be gone.

While these tests come suddenly and unexpectedly to our outer awareness, I believe that in our higher consciousness we know ahead of time what our tests in life will be and that we have been prepared for them in the heaven-world. God wants us to pass our tests, and he conspires with our Higher Selves to give us the best possible preparation for them. We carefully choose our families and circumstances in life before we take embodiment, and angels rehearse with us the tests we will have to pass and the tools we will need.

I believe that I was prepared for this test in many ways: through my work as a doctor, in my experiences as a minister, and in the work I did with others as they passed through their tests. Maybe that is why I got so involved in the life of my patient Cheryl and what she was experiencing. Perhaps my Higher Self was whispering to me, "Pay attention, because you will need to know about this one day." At a soul level, I believe I knew that I would also one day have to walk the same path that Cheryl did. Knowing her and helping her was a part of the preparation for my own healing journey.

An Initiation of the Heart

Within our body there are seven major energy centers, called chakras. These spiritual centers are aligned along the spinal column and are related to certain organs in the physical body. When energy is out of balance or not flowing correctly in the spiritual centers of the body, it can manifest as different kinds of imbalances, eventually resulting in illness or imbalance in the corresponding organs. Since the breast is close to and associated with the heart chakra, breast cancer can be seen to be related to this chakra.*

The heart chakra is the center of divine love, and the light of

---

* For further explanation of the chakras, see Appendix A, "Spiritual Anatomy."

this chakra at spiritual levels is a beautiful rose-pink. The heart chakra is often likened to a rose—a twelve-petaled rose-colored center from which divine love flows. Much has been written about the heart and the path of the heart. Even in our everyday language, the significance of the heart is seen: "A broken heart," "It pains my heart," "Get to the heart of the matter," "Follow your heart." These are but a few of the phrases that tell us that we all know intuitively how important the heart is.

The heart is our most important spiritual center. There is a spiritual flame that burns in your heart, and this light in your heart is greater than all of the darkness that is in the world. This is why the Bible says, "Greater is he that is in you, than he that is in the world."[2] The "he that is in you" is the spirit of the living God, the flame of life that is anchored within your heart.

For some time prior to my diagnosis, I had felt a pain in my heart. I had been greatly burdened in my work and by changes that had been occurring in the organization where I served. My spiritual teacher had been diagnosed with an incurable illness, the organization was in transition, and I cared deeply about many situations that I seemed to be unable to do anything about. I felt all of this as a pain in my heart.

This pain felt like a piercing of the heart, almost as if it were being pierced by a dagger. I could also feel it as a weight, heaviness, or burden around the area of the heart. I had felt this from time to time in my life, but never for such a prolonged period of time without respite and never with the feeling of being so powerless to lift the burden or do anything about it.

I had a dream where my heart was pierced by two spears. I could now relate to those pictures of Mary where her heart is pierced with a sword or surrounded by a crown of thorns. Although not brought up Catholic, I had accompanied some of my Catholic friends from medical school to Mass; I was familiar with the paintings of the pierced heart, although at the time it was hard for me to relate to those paintings of Mary. With the diagnosis of breast cancer, I felt that there was indeed someone in heaven who understood intimately the spiritual initiation that I have come to associate with breast cancer.

At the time, I wrote in my journal about the pain in my heart that was not a physical pain. Here is what I said:

I have watched two videos about Padre Pio. I pray to him and find it very helpful. He always told people to "pray, hope, and don't worry," which I find very comforting. He suffered so much and yet helped so many people—so many cures and miracles.

I feel quite well except for some loss of appetite and a pain in my heart that is not physical. The pain comes and goes. It eases when I pray and do spiritual work. When I think about my illness or sadness or dying or work or other stressful matters, the pain comes to my heart, and it extends into my right breast. It surely shows the mind-body connection. It is like someone literally pulling at my "heart-strings."

I am very focused in doing what I need to do for me. I am not able to help others right now and must keep silent and concentrate on myself. People who are depressed or not interested in my welfare burden me, and I feel it in my heart. Conversations with difficult people have made me realize that I need to work on forgiveness and hardness of heart.

I know that not every woman with breast cancer will feel this experience as I felt it, but I write of it because there will be those who will understand and for whom it will resonate with their own experience. If they read this story, they can know that they are not alone.

My experience as a minister, doctor, and patient tells me that breast cancer is an initiation of the heart chakra. It is a time of testing of the heart and the correct use of the energies of the heart. It is an initiation of love. No matter how much we love or have loved, it is a calling to come up higher and to love as never before.

It is a calling to a more spiritual love—not a co-dependent, sentimental or sympathetic love, but a deeper and truer love. That love might mean letting go of a part of our body or even our mode of life as we have known it. It may even mean the loss of our life altogether. All of these things, if we pass through them with grace, may be a means for the healing of the soul.

The first person I had to learn to love was myself. I found within me a love that was yearning to be expressed as greater care and nurturing of myself at all levels—physical, mental, emotional, and spiritual. I had to learn to love and not to fall into anger or bitterness or sadness or depression or hopelessness. I had to learn to love through the pain and turn the pain into bliss—the bliss of greater love for God and of my fellow man and woman. I had to learn to share greater love with others, whether they understood me or not. I saw this love as the love of Christ and his disciples, the love of the Holy Spirit that we all share.

THE LESSONS OF ILLNESS

I believe that all forms of cancer and, indeed, all life-threatening illnesses have a similar kind of spiritual lesson to share. Sometimes a clue to the specific lesson can be found in the location in the body or the nature of the illness. Sometimes it can be found through prayer and meditation. If you want to know, it is important to ask the questions:

What is the lesson here?

Is there something God could not show me any other way?

What do I need to do in order to pass this test?

And then be ready to hear the answers, and to make the necessary changes.

Sometimes we only find out what it was all about in retrospect. Some years after my experience with cancer I was speaking with my father-in-law about his. Thirty years earlier he had a very serious form of cancer, one that is nearly always fatal. The doctor told him to get his affairs in order. Surgery caused the left size of his face to be extremely disfigured. He could no longer work in his profession. But despite the doctor's prognosis of a year or two to live, three decades later he was still alive, although dealing with the effects of cobalt radiation. In spite of all that had happened, he said of his experience, "It taught me how to live."

I was acutely aware that I was not alone in my initiation. In fact, within 48 hours of my diagnosis, the realization came of how many other women were going through this illness at the same time. It staggered me. Here I was, going through this terrible thing, and thousands of others were going through it with me. I felt a great love and kinship for them. Why didn't someone tell me this was happening? Why hadn't I understood before this that one in eight women will experience breast cancer at some point in life? Why don't we teach every girl and teenager and woman how to prevent breast cancer? Why aren't we shouting it from the rooftops?

I was not alone. Many women had gone through breast cancer before me, and sadly, many would follow. I wanted to learn from those who had experienced it, and I wanted to share what I would learn with those who would come after me.

THE BODY OF THE MOTHER

I feel a oneness with all women who are suffering from breast cancer, and I feel that the heart of the Mother is one with all of us. We speak of Mother Earth, and in some nations people speak of their country as Mother, as in Mother Russia. Native Americans believe that we are all a part of Mother Earth. Hindus and Buddhists know many manifestations of the Divine Mother—Kali, Lakshmi, Durga, and Kuan Yin, to name just a few. We can even think of the entire physical universe as the manifestation of God as Mother, *Mater, Matter.*

I believe that we are all the body of the Divine Mother. There is the energy of Mother in our soul, our spirit, and our body, and whether we occupy a male or female body in this life, our physical body temple is the body of the Mother.

Today we are in an age when the light of the Divine Mother is intended to rise again, in the planet and in each one of its people. As this light rises, it activates many things, and we are collectively dealing with the effects of this light coming to the fore. We have to deal with the consequences of our individual and collective misuse of that light. This is a personal karma as well as a planetary karma, and its weight is something that we bear spiritually, even in our physical body.

Therefore, I ask myself the following questions:

Is not our Mother Earth suffering from all kinds of abuse?

Is not the heart of the Divine Mother weeping for her children during these troubled times?

Have we not seen the appearances of the Divine Mother in the person of Mary, as she has asked us to pray for her children?

And as we are one in the heart of the Divine Mother, especially those who wear feminine bodies in this life, perhaps our own spiritual hearts are also burdened—for one another and for our planet and her people—when we know that things are not as they should be, either in our own bodies or the body of Mother Earth. Perhaps it is no accident that so many women are suffering from this disease (dis-ease).

THE EXPERIENCE OF THE DARK NIGHT

I do not think that my experience is in any way unique—it is perhaps more common than we realize. Many people throughout the ages, men and women, all types of people, including saints and mystics, have borne illnesses in their bodies. Some bore their personal karma in the form of illness: they took that energy into their body and transmuted it through the suffering of the illness. Others have taken illness into their bodies as a means of balancing planetary karma—the sins of the world, if you will. They have also felt the piercing of the heart. Some of them have written of this experience.

With this initiation of the heart comes an experience that has been described as a "dark night." The sixteenth-century mystic Saint John of the Cross wrote about this initiation, which often comes to the soul in the form of serious illness or trial. John of the Cross describes two different dark nights that the soul experiences in the return to God—the dark night of the soul and the dark night of the Spirit.[3]

The dark night of the soul is when the soul is beset by its own karma. It is a period of darkness, when everything looks black. There may be a sense of depression or despair. Hopelessness and grief may burden the soul. This dark night may be triggered by an experience that life brings to us, such as the loss of a loved one, an accident or a serious illness, a painful relationship or a failed relationship, emotional or mental trauma, very difficult circumstances in life, or sudden loss of income. All kinds of things can trigger this deep grief, depression, and sense of darkness.

Most of us have experienced some element of the dark night of the soul at some time in our lives; there are few who have not been touched by some deep sadness or burden. Even living in a family where we are not understood or appreciated can be experienced as a dark night.

The dark night of the soul is experienced as one encounters the return of his or her personal karma. For a time, the human creation almost completely obliterates the light of the Higher Self. It is as if a dark cloud descends, and all appears to be dark and gloomy and devoid of light. One barely finds anything good or lovely upon which to dwell.[4]

I think most cancer patients experience these feelings at some time during their illness. In the experience of the dark night, the soul may also feel a sense of separation from God. The heavens seem closed, and prayers don't seem to go anywhere. For those who have a strong belief system, this can be a real test of faith, but many do emerge stronger spiritually from it.

The dark night of the Spirit is a different initiation—it is more intense and more severe. It occurs in the midst of the initiation of the crucifixion. (Jesus demonstrated this initiation for us publicly and tangibly, but many others have also passed through the same initiation spiritually in one form or another.) The dark night of the Spirit is when the soul is actually cut off completely for a period of time from God and the Higher Self. During this time we are required to sustain our connection to God through the light we have internalized within us. It was at this point on the cross that Jesus cried out, "My God, my God, why hast thou forsaken me?"[5]

As we go through the initiation, our loved ones and caregivers stand by and comfort us, yet they are not able to take us down from that cross. How often have I seen family members, especially mothers and fathers, say that they would gladly give their own lives for the life of their child, yet they could not. The initiation must run its course, even as the angels stand by to comfort the one who is on the cross and those who keep the vigil.

One may experience the initiation of the dark night of the soul several times in a lifetime; the initiation of the dark night of the Spirit generally comes only once. Either initiation may last from hours to days or months. Some may even undergo the test for years, and it may take on a variety of forms. Illness in all of its forms, particularly cancer and terminal illnesses, can be a crucifixion. Even the forms of cancer treatment, such as chemotherapy, can feel like a crucifixion. I certainly felt that sense of separation at times during chemotherapy. I believe that many who suffer in this way would be greatly comforted if they knew about the initiation of the dark night of the soul and dark night of the Spirit, and if they knew that "this too shall pass."

When we are on the cross with our Lord, time seems to stand still. We can see no light at the end of the tunnel, and it seems as if we will never be taken down. In addition, we feel powerless to help ourselves. We cannot even wipe our own face. It is then that we need others, when we require the prayers and ministrations of our loved ones and community.

What helps during these times? First, it helps to know that all things come to an end. The dark night does not last forever. Beyond the night is the resurrection and the new dawn.

Second, we can understand that suffering is one way in which we can balance karma. Saint Paul spoke of it as a means of earning a "better resurrection" (Hebrews 11:35). It can be a means of purifying and raising the soul.

I believe that surgery itself can also be a quick way to deal with personal karma. By willingly sacrificing a part of our physical being, we may also let go of an unhealthy portion of our spiritual being, opening a door to healing at other levels.

Friends and family may bring great comfort. If they can wipe our face and comfort us or help us carry some of the burden of the cross, this is surely a grace. However, we must play our part, too, and not leave it all up to others. (Most cancer patients that I have known do everything they can to carry the load, and the problem is more often not knowing how to allow others to help them.)

Even if we see ourselves going through a spiritual dark night, it does not mean we should reject modern methods of alleviating suffering, such as pain medication and all of the benefits of allopathic and complementary medicine. These are gifts of God for us, and we are intended to use them. There is no benefit in suffering needlessly when an alternative is available. Better to control the pain and do as much as we can with our lives.

Oil of spikenard can help ease the pain of the dark night. Spikenard was the oil that Mary Magdalene used to anoint Jesus in preparation for his crucifixion. This holy oil can help us through the initiations of the crucifixion, the resurrection, and the ascension.

But probably the greatest assistance and the greatest need is prayer and spiritual work. "Pray for one another, that ye may be healed. The effectual fervent prayer of a righteous man availeth much."[6] Prayers by the patient and prayers for the patient can make a great difference. I look forward to the day when every hospital and place of healing will be filled with prayer. Imagine hospitals with teams of people who pray for healing of body, mind, and spirit, for the alleviation of pain, depression, and complications of treatment, for divine direction for the staff and the patients, and for new methods of treating the diseases that are causing so much grief.

The use of the violet flame can also be a great assistance. The spiritual energy of this flame can help to lift physical, emotional, mental, and spiritual burdens and lighten our karmic load. The violet flame has its own intelligence, and it knows where to go and what to do. Anyone can use it. A simple prayer or mantra is all it takes to release the energy of the violet flame through the power of your Higher Self.

HEALING THE SPIRITUAL BODY

I approached my illness from the perspective of each level of our being—physical, emotional, mental, and spiritual. Although the physical body is the one we are most familiar with, these other components of our being have their own "bodies" through which they function. Thus, we also have an emotional body, a mental body, and an etheric or spiritual body (also known as the memory body). These bodies are interpenetrating forcefields, the vehicles that we occupy to experience life on planet Earth.

Those with spiritual sight tell us that illness first begins in the etheric body. It can often be seen there before it cycles through the mental body and the emotional body, finally manifesting in the physical body as the last stage in the process. By the time an illness becomes physical, it has most likely been with us a long time. If illness can be healed in any of the other three bodies before it reaches the physical body, then the physical disease may be totally averted before it ever materializes. Similarly, if we do have a physical condition, if we can heal the underlying causes in the finer bodies, this healing can also cycle in to the physical body. Most effective of all is to work on all levels simultaneously, and to do this we need to be able to work on health at a spiritual level as well as a physical one.

It is in the etheric body that the blueprint for life is written and stored. The other three bodies ultimately manifest the blueprint that is set here. So, it all starts here with the etheric body, and it is spiritual tools that are the key to healing this body.

We can give the etheric body what it needs by giving devotion and adoration to the source of life within us each day. We can realize that all healing ultimately comes from God, the creator of all life (by whatever name we might know this universal principle). I think of the divine physician Jesus and his saints in heaven.

We can consciously connect with that source of light and healing. Give glory and praise to God for his grace in our lives. Spend time each day meditating, praying, or communing with your divine source, the mighty Presence of God above you, and send love to that God-source. Many times you may even feel the waves of love on the return current— or in the events of your life and of the lives of the people around you.

We can send light and healing energy into the etheric body just as we do into the physical body for physical healing, into the emotional body for healing of emotional problems and wounds, and into the mental body for healing of our mind and psychology. Specifically, we can direct the violet light and the healing green light into the etheric body in order to restore the original, perfect pattern for all of the four lower bodies.

THE EQUATION OF KARMA

I know from experience that karma has an important role in our lives. It probably affects us more on a daily basis than we realize, and it is intimately connected to our spiritual initiations. I felt that karma could be a part of my experience with breast cancer—not the whole cause, but a part of it. I had the definite feeling that I had been down this road before, and I used to wonder if I had had this experience in a past life.

I have always enjoyed reading about karma and its relationship to disease. One fascinating source was the work of Edgar Cayce, who was known as the Sleeping Prophet and was one of the first well-studied medical intuitives. While in a trance state, he would reveal details of a patient's illness and what could be done to treat it. He diagnosed illnesses with astonishing accuracy and prescribed medical treatments that were years ahead of his time, often curing people with life-threatening diseases. Very often he would speak of the past life experience that contributed to the illness or the lessons that needed to be learned in this life.[7]

Other physicians have a similar understanding. Dr. Gladys McGarey, a student of Edgar Cayce, is internationally known for her work in holistic and integrative medicine. In her book *The Physician within You,* she tells of a patient with chest pain that defied diagnosis for years. The pain was severe and distracting, but all tests had failed to reveal anything and no doctor was able to help him. Dr. McGarey knew that the pain was real and asked her patient to keep a written record of his dreams. Although skeptical, he did, and sure enough, one dream had an interesting tale to tell.

He dreamed he was in the crusades, hundreds of years ago. He and his companions were charging an enemy fortification and met resistance when a spear pierced his armor and went into his chest. Dr. McGarey described the look of pain in his eyes when recalling the experience, and she told him he would have to forgive and forget, then forgive himself for the grievance that he bore so close to his heart. The patient understood, and she knew that the physician within would take it from there.[8]

I could understand such emotional pain. When I looked at my former patient Cheryl, I had felt as if I were looking at myself. She had pain in her heart that was not physical, and I felt while I was treating her that I knew what it was like to walk where she walked. I did not know at the time how close to the truth this was.

Several years after I completed my own treatment for breast cancer, God showed me an amazing thing: I had a gradual but vivid recall of a past life. I was shocked when it first happened, and it took me some days to come to grips with the experience.

I lived in rural England several hundred years ago. In those days, women had few options, and most of them revolved around a good marriage and children. Your station in life was your destiny, and if you were not born into the right station, you had little chance of any other type of fulfillment.

I was sad about circumstances in life that I could not control. I fell in love, but the man was of a different social class. His family intervened and cut off the relationship. Determined to marry only for love, I turned down all other suitors. I now faced a life of loneliness and near poverty, and I wondered about having made the right choice.

I could not find an outlet for my creative talents, and the creativity that I did express was not recognized beyond a small family circle. I developed breast cancer in my forties, the same age I developed cancer in this life, and died in great sadness and with a deep sense of grief and unfulfillment. I believe that my father in that life was also my father in this life. As often happens, we return to work again with those with whom we have a common destiny or to whom we owe a debt.

I think that perhaps God did not reveal this to me before I completed my treatment because I had enough to handle simply dealing with the breast cancer itself. It would not have helped to know in my outer mind that I had died as a result of breast cancer in a previous life. He wanted me to get through it and come out on the other side before showing me what my soul and Higher Self already knew.

As a spiritual counselor, I do not recommend that people try to contact their past lives. I believe that the veil is drawn over those experiences for good reason. Firstly, it is hard enough to deal with this life without dealing with memories from past lives. In most cases, it would simply be confusing and troublesome. Secondly, once we are aware of the past-life memory, then the karma of that lifetime is opened, and it may be too much for us to bear. Our karma normally returns to us in gradual increments to be balanced on a day-to-day basis, and it can be unwise to attempt to accelerate that process.

Another reason why it is not recommended to seek out memories of past lives is that a recall we may have or something that is told to us about a past life may not be accurate. We may think we did some terrible thing and be burdened by it when we did not do it at all. Conversely, we may mistakenly think we achieved great things and do not have to work so hard this time around.

In the end, the past is only prologue. We cannot rest on the laurels of past good works or be burdened or held back by past mistakes. What matters is what we do in this life, the one we have now.

Nevertheless, when we are ready for the memory, and if it will help us make progress on our spiritual path, our Higher Self may reveal a past-life experience. Until then, it is best not to pry. Normally, I would not share such an experience with others, but I do so here because I think that it illustrates an important point.

More and more people are having recall of their past lives. More and more people understand the truth of karma and reincarnation because they feel the movement of the stream of life within them. These things are not unlikely. We have all been a part of many events have happened in the history of the earth.

I believe that one seed of my breast cancer was causes I may have set in motion a long time ago in a past life, and I suspect that it goes even beyond that one life of which I am aware. God did not let me see the record until I was past the initiation and had overcome it. Yet, my soul knew and was preparing for it.

Did I cause my cancer? No, I do not believe that I did. However, once I had it, I was accountable and responsible for doing the best that I could to overcome it.

Did any one thing cause my cancer? Although there may be things that contributed to my developing cancer, I am not aware of any one thing that I did or did not do that caused it.

Was God punishing me? No. God is a loving God and he does not send punishments (although he may send us lessons to help us learn). Karma is not punishment. It is a teacher. God allows our karma to descend to teach us lessons that we may not be able to learn any other way.

Could I do something about it once I had it? Yes, and I did many things to help my body overcome the cancer.

Could I have prevented it? I could certainly have done some things that would have made it less likely, but I am not sure that these things would have prevented it. I believe that it was a life experience and a life lesson that I had to go through. Having had cancer twice, I am now doing many things that will, by the grace of God, make the recurrence of cancer less likely.

Having seen the record of a past life, it was very easy for me to recognize these same feelings in my present life, and I was facing similar tests again. This time I had the good karma to be happily married and to have found the love that had eluded me in the past. I also had a good career this time around. Yet, life was again presenting me with circumstances that I could not control, and I was not doing the things that I loved to do.

How was I going to handle it this time? Would I submit to the grief and hopelessness? Would I continue to allow circumstances to control my life? Or would I fight for my life and make the interior changes that would get me through the test? Would I learn to love in spite of the pain?

In many ways, breast cancer was a déjà vu experience. As I was going through my treatment, I already knew the pain and what it felt like to die of this condition. When the initiation was upon me, I paid close attention to the lessons, spiritual and material, that I would have to learn and pass through. I worked hard. I fought and did not give up, even though I was often assailed by depression and sadness. I applied everything that I had learned from my parents and my teachers and from life. I applied all that I had learned as a doctor to my condition and its treatment. I applied all that I had learned as a minister on the spiritual path. This time, by the grace of God, I tried to learn the lessons that cancer had to teach me. And this time, I believe I passed this test, and I believe that it is indeed by His grace.

One of the key lessons that I learned is that what happens to you is not as important as your reaction to it. I cannot control all of the circumstances in my life, but I can choose what I will do and what my path will be. Although I may pass through grief and sadness, I do not have to dwell in them or let them overtake me. I found out that I have far more control over things than I realized, if I could simply let go of the sense of needing to control. I am learning in a deeper way to surrender all things to God and to my Higher Self. For if I get my lower self out of the way, my Higher Self can act in its place.

An important lesson was to set loving boundaries. Cancer forced me to delineate what was me and what was not me. Here was this foreign thing invading my body—and like it or not I had allowed it. I learned to remove it with the help of medicine and the mind and the spirit. I changed my thoughts and my feelings, and I changed my life.

Just as I set loving boundaries in my body, I likewise set loving boundaries in my life. I learned to say no to things that do not feel right or are not my concern. I learned to take less responsibility for others and more for myself. And I learned a greater appreciation of the healing power of love. Although I knew it and practiced it before my illness, I understand it at a far deeper level now.

No matter what else happens in my life after cancer, I know that I have passed a major hurdle. Whether the cancer is gone for good or returns one day is not the central issue. I am a different person now. Having had and overcome cancer affects everything else I do and say and think. I have a greater sense of hope and love in my heart. I have a better relationship with everyone, including myself. I have a deeper relationship with God. I strive to do the best that I can for myself, and I seek ways to help others as best as I can.

WHAT CAN I LEARN FROM MY ILLNESS?

Cancer can be a teacher to our souls—a means of spiritual initiation and soul testing. Aside from being healed of cancer, learning the spiritual lessons may be the most valuable part of the journey through cancer. Here are a few questions that may help bring those lessons into focus.

Reflect on them, write about them in your journal, or talk about them with a counselor or supportive friend:

In what ways are my priorities and outlook on life different as a result of this experience?

What parts of the body or organs are involved in my condition? What does this symbolize for me?

What is the real lesson here for me?

Is there something God could not show me any other way?

What do I need to do in order to pass this test?

CHAPTER 17

RELATIONSHIPS AND HEALING

If you are blessed to be able to overcome cancer, you will find that you do not conquer it alone. I was, and am, greatly blessed in the network of friends in heaven and on earth who were assisting me. The angels and masters in heaven were a wonderful source of support, and I tugged upon their garments every day. I would recommend that anyone facing any challenge in life, whether cancer or any problem, do the same. Get to know your heavenly friends and talk to them often.

God also has those who serve as his hands and feet on earth. My earthly friends were a wonderful support system. Their prayers, smiles, and words of encouragement meant so much.

FAMILY AND FRIENDS

It is well known that patients who have the support of family, friends, and loved ones do better in their treatment and recovery. My own friends and family will probably never fully know what their support meant to me during some very dark hours.

Different people have different approaches, and some people like to keep serious health challenges to only a small circle of close friends and family. However, I decided to not hide my illness. I let everyone know what I was dealing with, and I wanted to be as truthful as possible. I also set some guidelines so that they would know how to help me. I asked them to be upbeat and positive with me when we met. I had enough depression of my own to cope with, and I did not need the burden of others feeling sorry for me. Genuine compassion was always welcome.

There were often times when I needed to be alone, but there were also times when I needed company. Just going shopping with a friend or taking time to share a cup of tea could brighten my day and my outlook. I kept all the cards, letters, and e-mails of support and reread them from time to time to remind myself of the love and prayers that people sent my way.

PATIENTS WHO HAVE THE SUPPORT OF FAMILY, FRIENDS, AND LOVED ONES DO BETTER IN THEIR TREATMENT AND RECOVERY.

One friend sent me a pillow for the bath along with bath oil and other things to pamper myself. Another sent me a box of videos to watch while going through my treatments—golden oldies, musicals, and other fun shows. And another friend and her teenage daughters sent a Pooh Bear Treasure Chest full of goodies. These unexpected gifts always lifted my spirits.

Another source of comfort and support was sharing stories with others who had either gone through or were going through the cancer experience. Every story was different, and I had an insatiable desire to know the stories of others. I loved to talk to other patients at the hospital.

ANGELS AMONG US

Some years ago, I was given a CD called *A Country Christmas*. There was one song that really moved me. It was called "Angels among Us" and spoke about the angels who come into our lives, seemingly out of nowhere, to help us through our "darkest hours."

There were many such "angels" who helped me during my illness. One was a security guard named Leo who worked at the hospital. Before my surgery, Peter and I were sitting late one night in the solarium on the fifth floor. It was during that period of "not knowing": we did not know what stage the cancer was, whether I would need to have a mastectomy, whether I would need chemotherapy or what that would entail. I was trying to be positive and at the same time realistic and was alternating between hope and despair.

Leo was making his rounds, dressed in his blue uniform. He stepped into the solarium, saw us sitting there and stopped to chat. He said, "What are you two kids up to?" We were a bit older than his children, and he took kind of a fatherly approach to us. It was good to talk about ordinary things and not just cancer, although cancer was never far from my mind. Somehow the conversation got around to prayer and how good God is.

I explained to Leo that I had felt led to this particular hospital. He assured me that I had come to the right place and told me how much he loved working there. The next night he was there again, and this time I asked him to pray with me, which he did.

Leo continued to take a genuine interest, and when I returned to the hospital for chemotherapy, he would often seek me out and drop in for a chat. I looked forward to those visits very much. He had been a patient at the hospital himself and knew how it felt to be very ill. He had a great sense of faith and had lived his life by it.

One night on about day four of the first round of chemotherapy, I was feeling absolutely awful. I did not realize it at the time, but I was reacting to the drugs Compazine and Reglan, given to allay the nausea and vomiting. They worked for the nausea, but the side effects were beginning to compound. I started to get severe symptoms.

Leo stopped by and we talked about spiritual things, and the conversation turned to the crucifixion and what Jesus had gone through. I was becoming very distressed and asked Leo to pray for me. He held my hand and said a beautiful prayer that helped a lot.

I remember thinking that we all have times when we need help. Jesus could not do anything for himself while he was on the cross. Even while he was carrying his cross, Veronica had to wipe his face and Simon the Cyrenian had to help him carry it. And so it is that when we face big challenges in life, we can be a Veronica or a Simon to one another.

I knew that God was working through Leo that day. I believe that part of the spiritual initiation of cancer is a sense of hopelessness whereby we are humbled. We come to learn that we need others, and if we can allow them to help us, we will be greatly blessed. This is not always easy for people who are used to looking after others.

The kindness of people never ceased to amaze me. For months I could not wear mascara, as my eyes would fill with tears whenever someone was kind to me. I often felt that God was trying to tell me how much he loved me and cared for me through the kindness of friends and strangers, and I felt my heart opening.

Another embodied angel was Percy McCray, co-director of pastoral care and one of the hospital chaplains. Percy has a great laugh, a wonderful smile, an enthusiasm for life, and a love of people that is infectious.

I kept hearing about Percy from other patients, and though I wanted to meet him, we never could seem to connect. One day he came to visit another patient in my room while I was receiving chemotherapy. After he finished talking with her, I grabbed his hand and jokingly said, "Percy, this is my third visit to the hospital, and I still have not met you. I am not going to let you leave until you talk to me."

He chuckled and sat down, and we talked. He gave me some healing affirmations from the Bible. Before he left, he asked if he could pray with us, then gave the most beautiful and powerful prayer. You could feel the energy in the room shifting. Peter and I looked at each other after Percy left and said to one another, "Now that man has the Holy Spirit."

Percy's services every Wednesday morning at the hospital were a joy. We patients would come, pulling our intravenous equipment with us, still attached to the chemo. I always came away uplifted. Two of his sermons were "Faith, the Breakfast of Champions" and "Have You Got the Right Stuff?" (His answer was, *of course* we have the right stuff—because we all have *God* in us.)

There are many other friends and fellow patients I have met whose stories have touched my heart. There are some whose names I do not remember but whose faces I cherish—those who shared their stories with me, some who are winning the fight against cancer, and some who are not. I believe that though some may have lost in the outer sense, they have yet won an inner battle.

RETURNING TO ZION

Meeting these people is one reason I keep going back to the hospital in Zion, Illinois, for my checkups. They have excellent medical and alternative care, and there is a loving, supportive staff and community. But beyond all this, there are other things that I need to be reminded of periodically.

Zion is the name of the hill in Jerusalem where Solomon's Temple was built. It is the place where God is with his people and the place where we go to be with God. When I go to Zion, once again I can come apart and ponder the meaning of the illness that I once had. Once again, I become a patient. I submit to the tests and I humble myself to be a "patient one," waiting with fellow patients to have our tests and to be evaluated.

It is an opportunity to return to the center of my life and reassess. How am I doing? What is really important in my life? Am I where I need to be in body, mind, and spirit?

Being among fellow cancer patients, I am reminded that cancer can return, and that is a humbling thought. I am reminded of my mortality. The body is a vehicle for the Spirit, and I need to take care of my body in order to fulfill my purpose for being here.

I am reminded of the need to take care of first things first and to live each day as it comes to the best of my ability. I am reminded of the things that are important—family, friends, and relationships, my relationship to God, and how God works through others.

I also need the opportunity to share my story so that other patients can see someone else who has "gotten through chemo." As I hear the stories of others and see their fight, I remember my own. I need to be reminded of what it takes to win the fight.

THE RELATIONSHIP WITH OUR HIGHER SELF

One of the most important relationships that we can nurture is the relationship with our Higher Self. This is something I worked on diligently during my cancer treatment.

There are many names for this Higher Self. I understand it as the best and highest part of our being. It is the part of us that was born as pure spirit in the heart of God. In the East, they speak of the Buddha-nature or the *atman*. Christian mystics from the time of Saint Paul have spoken of the individualization of the Christ—"until Christ be formed in you."[1] This is the being of which John spoke as the individualized presence of the Son of God, "the true Light, which lighteth *every* man that cometh into the world."[2] Some think of the Higher Self as the inner teacher, the divine spouse, the dearest friend. Some recognize it as guardian angel.

I see this beloved one as just above me, overshadowing me, available to help me at any hour of the day or night. It manifests as the still small voice that speaks from within the heart and prompts me when I need help.

The relationship with my Higher Self requires work, just as any relationship does. There is a big difference between knowing about this relationship and actually engaging in it. As I went through my cancer treatment, I took the time for prayer and attunement with my Higher Self. And as I did so, I found a new centeredness. I felt I was becoming more of who I really am. If we draw close to our Higher Self, he will draw nigh to us.[3]

THE HEALING POWER OF FORGIVENESS

During my illness I came to understand anew the importance of forgiveness. I had always done my best to forgive and not hold onto old hurts or grudges, but a diagnosis of cancer makes one reassess everything. I realized I had to look at this area of my life again.

I asked myself some hard questions: Was there anyone in my life, past or present, whom I had not forgiven? Furthermore, was I able to forgive myself for my real or imagined shortcomings?

Sometimes I did not like what I saw. In some cases, I had withheld love and forgiveness. It was not that I hated or was angry or consciously not forgiving others, yet I was carrying around some baggage that I no longer needed, and I was not expressing the fullness of the love that I should have been expressing to all life—and to some people in particular.

I began to work diligently on this spiritual problem of non-forgiveness because I knew from my work as a minister that we pay a big price when we do not forgive. We pay the price with a lack of peace, with dis-ease in the mind and emotions, often contributing to disease in the physical body. It's simply enlightened self-interest to forgive.

Forgiveness follows spiritual law and principles, and all the great spiritual teachers have taught us to forgive. Forgiveness is the very first step on the spiritual path—unless we can forgive, we can make no real progress spiritually. And did you ever notice that Jesus often forgave people before he healed them? I was following a deep understanding that all healing begins with forgiveness. I wanted to follow in Jesus' footsteps; therefore, I had to be willing to forgive and be forgiven.

Within a few days of my diagnosis, I went to work and called each person who was a part of the team that I had worked with for the past two years and asked for their forgiveness for anything that I might have done, knowingly or unknowingly, that might have been a burden to them during our association.

Human relationships are often difficult. Sometimes when I asked for forgiveness, I discovered that there were indeed those whom I had wronged or hurt without realizing it.

A few months later, in May of 1999, I had a dream that taught me an important lesson about forgiveness. I dreamed about a person with whom I had worked closely for six months several years earlier. He and I had had some disagreements. We had several discussions where we shared our feelings, agreed to disagree, asked for forgiveness, and seemed to achieve a good resolution. I thought that we had resolved everything, yet my dream showed me that further resolution was needed. In the dream, he and I met in a dining room at a party. I came up to him and asked him for forgiveness, and he asked me for forgiveness. We then embraced, the room filled with violet light, and the negative energy between us lifted.

When I awoke, I was astounded at the dream. I thought that we had ended our relationship on good terms and that there was nothing unresolved between us. We had both understood the equation of karma in relationships and felt that perhaps the difficulties between us were the result of a past-life problem resurfacing. We had consciously approached the situation from the highest spiritual perspective of which we were capable, and we thought that it was done. However, I was not fully comfortable in his company and wondered if I was still harboring some resentment.

The dream prompted me to take further action. I consciously went back over our working relationship and released any energy that was tied up in it. I sent him love and gave mantras to the violet flame to transmute any negativity or karma between us.

I thought about talking to him but decided not to, because I really did not know how to broach the subject with him. But each morning, I would awake with the feeling that I needed to call him. Finally, after a few weeks, I did call and simply told him what had happened. I explained my dream and the prompting that I had to call him. I asked him to forgive me. He seemed surprised and asked, "For what?" He was not aware of any problem. Nevertheless, he said he would be happy to forgive me. We talked a little, and then the conversation was over.

Some months later, I saw him in a social setting. He came over, and this time he asked for forgiveness. Now I was taken aback—in fact, I was moved to tears. I have no idea what prompted him to do this, but of course, I gave him my forgiveness and we embraced, just as in the dream. This time I felt a difference. I felt that whatever problem we had between us from a past life was now finally resolved.

This experience taught me that forgiveness may be a process—it is like peeling an onion, there are layers and layers. You peel one layer, you cry a little, and you think it is over; and then there is another layer.

I do not know why I needed to take the additional steps that I did in this case, and I do not think that he knew, either. I am not sure if it was for him or for me or for both of us, but I trusted in the dream. I also believe that the dream was a recall of an experience in the retreats of heaven. I was being shown that I needed to supply the unguent of the violet flame to the situation and to work on forgiveness. For whatever reason, it was necessary, and I was happy to follow the inner direction I had been given.

The following is a mantra that I gave each day when I felt that I needed to forgive and work on forgiveness. I would usually give it three or nine times. On occasion I would give it thirty-three times a day, as a Catholic would give a novena. It has a very soothing effect on the body, mind, and soul. As I gave it I would also visualize the violet flame surrounding myself and the person to whom I was sending forgiveness.

> I AM forgiveness acting here
> Casting out all doubt and fear,
> Setting men forever free
> With wings of cosmic victory.
>
> I AM calling in full power
> For forgiveness every hour;

To all life in every place,
I flood forth forgiving grace.[4]

Forgiveness is necessary not only for our individual healing but also for healing the planet. Psychotherapist and author Robin Casarjian explains this well in her book *Forgiveness: A Bold Choice for a Peaceful Heart.* She says, "Forgiveness is a required course for all of us. There is no way for us to have world peace without it. Forgiveness gives each of us the immediate power to play a vital and necessary part in a planetary peacemaking and evolutionary process. If enough individuals choose to live from their heart for more and more moments, perhaps we will reach that critical mass when world healing is not only possible, but inevitable."[5] When we look at the Middle East and other places where hatreds and anger go on for generation after generation, we can understand the truth of these concepts.

Hatred, anger, and non-forgiveness bind us to that which we hate. We separate ourselves from the presence of our Higher Self if we have withheld forgiveness from any part of life. By forgiving others and accepting forgiveness, we can actually free ourselves from many burdens of body, mind, and spirit.

KUAN YIN, BODHISATTVA OF COMPASSION

For anyone having difficulty with forgiveness, I recommend that you get to know Kuan Yin, the compassionate savioress from Chinese lore. She is known to Buddhists throughout Asia as the bodhisattva of compassion and the goddess of mercy.

I like to think of Kuan Yin as the Eastern version of Mary. She is much beloved of the common people, who give her prayers and mantras just as many people in the West love to give the rosary.

Kuan Yin calls us to ask for forgiveness even when we think that we have done nothing wrong. Ask, because it is a part of the code of heaven and because it gives the other person the opportunity to ask for forgiveness, too. It was because of Kuan Yin and her teaching that I asked everyone whom I knew for forgiveness—and this path led me where I never thought that it would.

Although she is a part of Eastern culture, Kuan Yin is becoming more known by devotees in the West for her compassionate heart and her ability to assist with difficult problems. If you would like to find out more about Kuan Yin, a great place to start is John Blofeld's book, *Bodhisattva of Compassion: The Mystical Tradition of Kuan Yin.* The book includes a number of very touching stories of Kuan Yin's intercession.

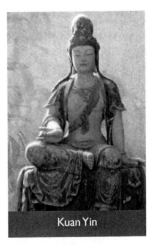

Kuan Yin

Kuan Yin has long had a special place in my heart. Her statues have graced my office and home for many years. Although she is depicted in many forms, she is most often portrayed as a white-robed goddess or a slender woman in flowing white robes who carries in her left hand a white lotus, the symbol of purity.

In Buddhist lore, Kuan Yin is known as a sponsor of children and families, and I had found in my medical practice that she is fantastic at helping women in labor or women who are trying to get pregnant. She is also an expert at dealing with tough situations where there seems to be no way out.

There are many tales I could tell of her intercession in my life. Some are too personal to share, but here is one example, a patient in my medical practice in Australia years ago.

It was one of those really busy days when I was overloaded and very stressed. My next patient came into the room, a pretty, petite Asian woman who spoke only a little English. She was not one of my regular patients. She brought her daughter with her, a lovely little girl about two years old. As her sad story unfolded, she started to cry, and her little girl was in tears too.

The woman was about fourteen weeks pregnant, but her husband was not the father of the child. She was unhappy in her marriage. Her husband was very strict and rarely showed affection, even though he loved her. She had a very brief affair, an ill-fated one-night liaison, while her husband was out of town on business. She regretted it immediately and never saw the man again. But much to her horror, she discovered she was pregnant.

She knew by her dates that her husband could not be the father. She was afraid that the child would look like the biological father— tall, blond, and blue-eyed. She also knew her husband would never understand—he would know that it was not his child and he would divorce her immediately.

It seemed unthinkable to have the baby. There was no other choice in her mind, although she did not like the concept of abortion. To make matters worse, she had taken a Chinese medicine to try to get rid of the baby, but it had not worked. Now she was worried that if she did keep the baby, it would be deformed or harmed in some way.

While she cried, we discussed all of her options in broken English. I sat with her, held her hand, listened, gave her a hug, and suddenly remembered Kuan Yin.

I usually never mention my spiritual beliefs to patients, but for some reason, I knew it was right to talk to this lady about Kuan Yin. I simply asked her if she believed in Kuan Yin. She was astounded that I knew about her and she stopped crying. Yes, she believed in Kuan Yin but had not prayed to her since her childhood. Her mother had been a devotee and had taught her the mantras.

I recited a mantra for her: CHIU K'U CHIU NAN P'U-SA LAI.* "Save from suffering, save from calamity, Bodhisattva—come!" She smiled, because this was the one her mother used.

Somehow things started to look up. I cannot explain why, as nothing had changed in her outer circumstances. She said she would think about things and she would come back to see me so we could talk further. She returned a couple of days later, totally changed. She had prayed to

---

* Pronounced: JEE-OH KOO JEE-OH NAHN POO-SAH LYE.

Kuan Yin and had decided to keep the baby. She had even had told her husband that she was pregnant. He was delighted and hoped for a son to carry on the family name. He did not ask any questions, and she never told him about the affair, as she felt that everything would turn out right.

She came to see me during the rest of the pregnancy, even though she lived some distance away, and she always gave me a big hug and a kiss when she saw me.

The birth itself was easy. It was a boy, and wonder of wonders, he looked just like her husband! Everyone remarked upon it. She came to see me one more time to thank me, but I told her to thank Kuan Yin. I never saw her again, and for a long time I kept the picture she gave me of her "miracle" baby.

Does it sound like a fantastic story? Not to a devotee of Kuan Yin.

I tugged often on Kuan Yin's white robe during my journey through cancer. For me, she has become the court of last resort: if no help seems to be forthcoming from any other master or angel in heaven, and things are looking grim, Kuan Yin is the one I go to. I gave her mantras each day during my treatment, using a beautiful recording called *Kuan Yin's Crystal Rosary*.

Early in my six weeks of radiation treatment, a friend sent me a glow-in-the-dark statue of Kuan Yin. Although this was half in jest, she also knew that I am very fond of Kuan Yin and that I would sincerely appreciate the gift. The statue made me smile. She was a comforting presence when I turned out the light at night. I could see her glowing silently in the dark and keeping watch over me. Though I am thankfully through the cancer experience, I still keep that statue by my bedside.

I believe that masters and angels can radiate light and healing through gemstones and crystals. They can also place their presence over their statues and pictures, which then become focuses of light; heavenly beings can actually radiate a light and a presence through these focuses when needed. I know that this happened for me during my treatment.

HEAVENLY HELPERS

The heaven-world has always been very real to me. From the time I was a child I have been comfortable with a heaven filled with angels, saints, and masters waiting to help us if we will simply invite them into our lives.

Many of those who have had near-death experiences have said that the heaven-world is even more real than the physical world in which we live. I spend a lot of my day as a minister and counselor working with that realm, and while we may not be able to see its inhabitants on a daily basis, they are standing just the other side of the veil, ready to help as much as they can. Some people do see them (including many who have gone through a near-death experience), but you don't need to see them to be able to work with them. The key is to know that they can help us most effectively if we ask for their assistance and work with them cooperatively.

There are specialists in heaven, just as there are specialists on earth. There are angels of protection, angels of healing, angels of love, and angels who can help us with our psychology. And when you need specific help, it is best to go to an expert.

One of these heavenly friends who gave me great comfort was the great Catholic saint Padre Pio. I read books about his life and watched videos of his healing ministry. This blessed saint knew great suffering while he lived, and he is well-known for performing miracles of healing—even more so now that he is in heaven.

I am also greatly devoted to Mary the mother of Jesus, who is known as Queen of the Angels. I gained great comfort from her presence as I gave her rosary each day. I like to think of Kuan Yin, Mother Mary, and other masters and saints as part of a heavenly team that helped me through my cancer treatment. I give much of the credit to them, because I feel that in the end, all healing comes from God.

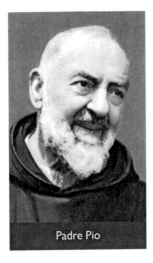

Padre Pio

PRAY, HOPE, AND DON'T WORRY!
—Padre Pio

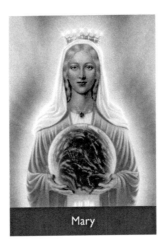

Mary

KEYS FOR HEALING THROUGH RELATIONSHIPS

✓ **Nurture your relationship with your Higher Self.**

✓ **Remember the important things in life—family, friends, and relationships.** God can work through friends and loved ones to bring comfort and support.

✓ **Share stories with others** who have gone through or are going through the cancer experience.

✓ **Forgive others and accept forgiveness.** This can free you from many burdens of body, mind, and spirit. Ask yourself:

    o Is there anyone in my life, past or present, whom I have not forgiven?

    o Am I able to forgive myself for my real or imagined shortcomings?

    o Can I take the next steps of forgiveness?

✓ **If forgiveness is difficult, invite heavenly helpers to assist you.**

CHAPTER 18

WOULD I DO IT ALL OVER AGAIN?

I have had a most amazing and blessed healing journey through breast cancer. When I was first diagnosed, I never would have thought that I would one day feel cancer was one of the best things that ever happened to me. I had heard other people say this in the past, and I could never really understand what they meant. I understand now.

The day after my first mammogram, when I knew that I had a suspicious lump but I did not yet know whether it was cancer, I saw a friend who is an astrologer. He pulled me into his office, called up my chart on his computer, and said, "This is a liberating time. Be yourself. It is an opportunity to express who and what you are and to become more of yourself. Set some limits. Deal with unresolved issues and impediments to your expression without masking or holding back who you are. Express your creativity. There is evidence of a struggle to find your identity and career. It is an opportunity for new friends and new expressions of self. Restructure and realign yourself. The hidden will come to the surface in the physical and emotional quadrants of your being. In summary, there is ample opportunity to break through if you do not lose sight of who and what you are."

As I look back on the experience, I can see that this was very accurate, and all that he said has come to pass. I was given a great opportunity to express who I am and become more of myself.

Don't get me wrong—I would not wish cancer on anyone, and I have no desire to go through the experience again. However, even though it was the most difficult thing that I have ever had to go through, I would not swap that experience for the world. Overcoming cancer is a part of the person I have become and who I am today. I can honestly say that I believe that I am a better and stronger person because of it.

Would I make the same choices again?

Given the same circumstances that I faced then—absolutely.

Would I expect others to make the same choices?

Not at all. Everyone is different, and no two cancers are the same. Each person must make his or her own choices.

Will I make the same choices in the future if I have to?

I cannot predict the future, and so I will wait and see. Like everyone who has faced cancer, I am aware that it could return. In fact, having had cancer twice before, I may be statistically more likely to have it again. On the other hand, I know that my life is vastly different now. I have made changes that helped me overcome cancer and also ones I hope will prevent cancer in the future.

PREVENTION IS BETTER THAN TREATMENT

Prevention is a whole lot better than treatment. Although I have no idea if my cancer was preventable, I certainly like to think that future cancers are preventable. I approach my life in that way.

Here are some of the ways I am working on prevention:
- Regular breast self-examination aimed at early detection
- Continued regular medical follow-up
- Use of complementary medical techniques
- Attention to nutrition and diet
- Regular exercise and movement, including breathing exercises

- Prayer and spiritual work
- Work on the mind-body connection
- Support and networking with friends who have had cancer

Like anyone who has had breast cancer, I pray that the cancer will not return, and I do the best I can to keep it out of my life by applying all that I have learned.

Having said that, if cancer were to resurface in my life, I would again carefully and prayerfully consider all of my options—from surgery and mastectomy to chemotherapy and radiation and all forms of complementary therapies. I would examine again even those options that I rejected before. For I am a different person now than I was then.

Having considered all my options, I would follow my heart and allow it to lead me to the right choices. I would also try to allow myself to be surprised, because truly, if you had told me while I was practicing medicine that I would one day put myself through chemotherapy, I would not have believed you.

Having gone through this experience, I feel a sense of responsibility to share what I have learned. Perhaps one reason I feel this keenly is because of a female health practitioner in our community years ago who had died of breast cancer after forgoing surgery and medical treatment and using only alternative therapies. She had wanted to cure her cancer naturally. Apparently it was a death that might have been prevented if she had considered surgery to remove the tumor.

I also knew of other women since that time who have died after making similar choices and some who had a lumpectomy but declined the radiation their doctors recommended, only to find that the cancer returned very quickly. These women seemed to have a misconceived idea that a spiritual approach to healing should use only alternative healing techniques and could not include regular medical care.

In my role as a doctor and minister, I sought to blend the two, and I hoped that others might benefit from what I learned.

If you are facing cancer, or if you know someone else who is, I would encourage you to do all that you can to meet this challenge on every level:

- Embrace it, face it, and don't ignore it.
- Pursue the best of all forms of treatment. Don't ignore traditional medical care.
- Look for alternatives, but be realistic about them.
- Think of cancer as a teacher and discover the lessons that it has to teach you.
- Take an honest look at your life and see if you are ignoring any of the laws of wholeness.
- Decide what is important from the perspective of the heart and make your decisions prayerfully.
- Love yourself and be kind to yourself and your body.
- Don't beat yourself up, but make the changes you can in your life.
- Reach out to those who love you, and love them back.
- Pray and ask others to pray for you.
- Pursue spiritual healing and put your inner doctor to work.
- Use spiritual techniques for healing, including the violet flame.
- Reach up to the Source of all life, and allow it to guide you.
- Fight hard, yet recognize the point where it is time to let go and let God act.
- Do the best that you can, and know that you are safe in God's hands.

Cancer is a subject that is very close to my heart. I have lived and breathed it, and at one stage in my life, it dominated my every waking thought and even my dreams. It became the central focus of my life at the time, but I felt that it needed to, because I was fighting for my life. I felt that I needed to do the things that I did, and I have no regrets.

This cycle of life now is behind me, and I have moved on to other assignments. If the cycle should come round again, I will fight again and fight hard, as long as God gives me breath. And if he should decide that it is time to take me home, I will embrace that decision too.

This is my personal healing journey through cancer. It may not be for everyone, but it was my way. If you are dealing with the challenge of cancer, I hope that in walking a while with me, you have felt that another person, just like yourself, has trod a similar path to the one you are now on. You, too, are on a journey. Allow it to take you where it leads you, to teach you what you need to know.

If you can use some or all of my experience and learn from it, this book will have achieved its goal.

I pray that you will have every good fortune and many victories on your own healing journey. With all my heart, I wish you Godspeed. I am praying for you and for all who read this book.

Neroli Duffy

CHECKLIST: PREVENTING CANCER OR ITS RECURRENCE

✓ Take care of your diet.

✓ Maintain your optimum weight.

✓ Exercise regularly.

✓ Find your goal in life and pursue it wholeheartedly.

✓ Find constructive ways to deal with stress.

✓ Learn to set loving boundaries,

✓ Forgive others and ask for forgiveness.

✓ Let go of negative emotions.

✓ Pray and develop your spiritual life.

✓ Use the violet flame to lighten your karmic load.

✓ Find ways to serve others.

✓ If you have had cancer, seek support and networking from other survivors.

✓ Have regular screening for early detection.

CHECKLIST: KEYS FOR FACING THE CHALLENGE OF CANCER

✓ Face it, embrace it—don't ignore it.

✓ Pursue the best of all forms of treatment. Don't ignore traditional medical care.

✓ Look for alternatives, but be realistic about them.

✓ See cancer as a teacher and discover the lessons that it has for you.

✓ Take an honest look at your life and see if you are ignoring any of the laws of wholeness.

✓ Decide what is important from the perspective of the heart and make your decisions prayerfully.

✓ Love yourself and be kind to yourself and your body.

✓ Don't be too hard on yourself, but make the changes you can in your life.

✓ Reach out to those who love you, and love them back.

✓ Pray and ask others to pray for you.

✓ Pursue spiritual healing and put your inner doctor to work.

✓ Use spiritual techniques for healing, including the violet flame.

✓ Reach up to the Source of all life, and allow it to guide you.

✓ Fight hard, yet know the point where it is time to let go and let God act.

✓ Do the best that you can, and know that you are safe in God's hands.

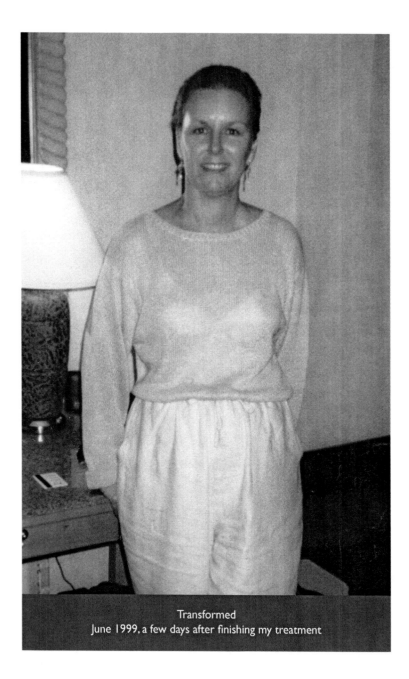

Transformed
June 1999, a few days after finishing my treatment

SPIRITUAL ANATOMY

In medical school I studied the anatomy of the human body in order to understand its function. When I began to study spirituality, I longed to know more about the anatomy of the spirit and how it meshed with the physical body, the mind, and the emotions. Here are some of the things that I learned—an abbreviated lesson in your spiritual anatomy.

The concepts are universal, and elements of them can be found in many different spiritual and religious traditions. Many of the specifics of the concepts described below I learned from the writings of Elizabeth Clare Prophet.

THE HIGHER SELF

Everyone has a Higher Self. We each have a unique spiritual destiny. One of the keys to fulfilling that destiny is recognizing that we have a divine nature and a direct relationship with God (by whatever name we might know that universal presence).

Our Higher Self is the source of the energy that keeps us going every day. The Higher Self is a powerhouse of light and energy that we can plug into and access for healing and wholeness.

Dr. Gladys Taylor McGarey wrote a book called *The Physician within You.* I like to think of my Higher Self as this doctor within. When I was practicing medicine, I sometimes received flashes of insight and intuition that enabled me to help my patients. When this happened, I believe that it was my Higher Self working with the Higher Self of the patient.

Our Higher Self is the true director of our healing and we can all tap into a higher source when we seek healing. This is the part of us that works with the angels who attend us, including our guardian angel. The Higher Self is sometimes called the Real Self, because it is actually more real than our physical body. It has a permanent existence, while our physical body lasts for only one lifetime.

Our Higher Self sees the big picture and knows the keys that will unlock the doors to our wholeness as well as the timetable for our healing. It tries to guide us and point us in the right direction, but sometimes we do not listen. It speaks through the still small voice within, and it gives unerring guidance in all things, small and great. Part of the healing process for many people is learning to listen again to that voice and to follow it. That is how illness can sometimes be a wake-up call—it causes us to stop, reassess, and go within. It impels us to go back and pick up those dropped stitches on the path of life, the things that we knew we should have done but somehow did not.

Some people who have had near-death experiences have seen this Higher Self. However, you don't have to die to see that Higher Self. Many saints and mystics have seen this vision, and they have described it in many different ways. Elizabeth Clare Prophet has depicted that Higher Self visually in her "Chart of Your Divine Self." She speaks of this chart as a portrait of you (the soul evolving in time and space, seen in the lower figure) and the God within you (seen as the upper figures).

The upper figure in the chart is your individual God-Presence, or I AM Presence,* the highest part of your being and the source from which your soul came forth to experience life in this world. The I AM Presence is surrounded by the causal body, seven spheres of light corresponding to the seven rays, the seven chakras, and seven qualities of the Christ consciousness. From the center to the periphery, the spheres are white

---

* The name of God as "I AM" was first given to Moses when he asked God to reveal his name. The response he received was, "I AM THAT I AM. Thus shalt thou say unto the children of Israel, I AM hath sent me unto you." [Exod. 3:14]

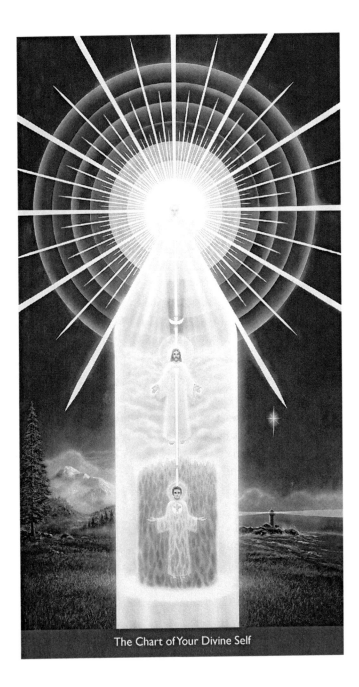

The Chart of Your Divine Self

in the center, the quality of purity; golden yellow, wisdom; pink, divine love; violet, freedom and transmutation; purple and gold; peace and service; green, healing; and blue, power, protection and the will of God.

The middle figure in the chart is the mediator between the upper figure (the pure perfection and intensity of light in the I AM Presence) and the lower figure (the soul evolving in the world). This mediator is the Christ consciousness, the individualized presence of the Son of God.

THE FOUR LOWER BODIES

Even though many people understand that they have a Higher Self, it is easy to get caught up with the physical body, not realizing that the body is simply the vehicle for the Spirit. In fact, the dimensions and all-ness of our Spirit cannot be contained within the physical form to which we are so attached.

When we are born, we are given a physical body that develops in the womb as a home for the Spirit. However, as well as a physical body, we also have our memories, mind, and emotions. These faculties are not dependent on the physical body, and each of these elements of our being is associated with what can be thought of as its own "body." Thus, the lower figure in the Chart of Your Divine Self is actually made up of four bodies: a memory body (or etheric body), a mental body, an emotional body, and a physical body.

These four bodies are interpenetrating sheaths of consciousness, each vibrating in its own dimension. They are the vehicles by which we experience the world of time and space and are known as the four lower bodies.

These bodies are intended to function as an integrated whole. Each body affects the others in different ways, and when there is a problem in one of the bodies, it can affect the others. The techniques of psychoneuroimmunology use these connections between the bodies by harnessing the mind and emotions to affect the immune system and the physical body.

In my healing journey, I tried to work on healing in each of the four lower bodies. For me, the real definition of health in body, mind, and Spirit is when the four lower bodies are all in sync and aligned with the blueprint of life that is held by the Higher Self.

SEVEN ENERGY CENTERS

The soul clothed in the four lower bodies is connected to the Higher Self by the stream of light that can be seen in the Chart of Your Divine Self. This thread of contact is known as the silver cord or the crystal cord. It is over this connection that we receive the light and energy of our Higher Self. The crystal cord is anchored in the body in the heart center, and from there this energy is distributed throughout the body via a network of spiritual centers known as chakras (a Sanskrit term for "wheel" or "disk").

These chakras regulate the flow of energy to different parts of your body. The seven major chakras are positioned along the spinal column from the base of the spine to the crown. Each chakra is a sending and receiving station for the particular quality of energy associated with that chakra. For example, the quality expressed through the heart chakra is love.

These spiritual centers are not static points of light but dynamic energy centers that constantly take in and send out spiritual light and energy. They are intimately connected to the health and vitality of the organs and parts of the body associated with them (see the chart at the end of this appendix). Hence, it is helpful to know about these centers and their functioning when seeking healing. In fact, many complementary therapies work directly with these spiritual centers.

The chakras go through an evolutionary process as we develop spiritually. They range from small and dormant to fully awakened, where they emit much light. These centers can look different in different people, depending on past and present use of energy and the spiritual development of the individual. They are the body's primary centers of the network of energy flow that is the focus of many alternative healing techniques.

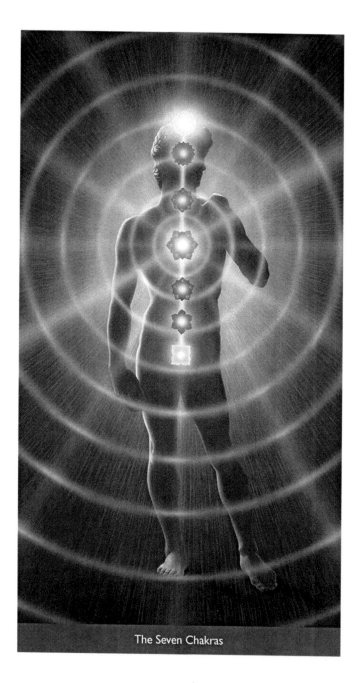

The Seven Chakras

The heart chakra is the most important spiritual center. It is related to the physical heart and the organs of the chest. I believe that breast cancer, in particular, is an initiation of the heart. This is the spiritual center that I worked with the most when I had cancer.

THE AURA

The correct care and use of these energy centers leads to greater vitality in our physical body as well as our three finer bodies as each chakra takes in and gives out energy according to its specific frequency.

As light streams forth from the chakras, it forms a radiating energy field, the aura, that penetrates and extends beyond the boundaries of the physical form. The size of the auric forcefield is directly related to the light that is anchored in the seven energy centers. Through the aura we each affect the world and the people around us, constantly sending out the vibration of that which is within.

Through the aura, we can also sense the vibrations of the world around us. Here's an example. You can walk into a room and often tell if someone is upset or unhappy, even if they give no outer sign of a problem. Likewise, you can also spot people who exude positive energy. We all love to be with people who make us feel better—their spirit is almost infectious. We also know those people who make us feel depressed every time we talk to them.

The aura is not static. It is constantly changing from moment to moment depending on the quality and vibration of thoughts and feelings. The aura also reflects the health and vitality of the physical body and all of the four lower bodies. In fact, the signs of disease are often found in the etheric, mental, and emotional bodies long before they appear physically, and those with spiritual sight may see those signs even before the physical manifestation.

Many spiritual healing techniques work at the level of the aura and the finer bodies. As healing and the flow of energy are restored at those levels, the healing can also follow on the physical.

CHAKRA	RELATED ORGANS OF THE PHYSICAL BODY
Base of the spine	adrenals
Seat of the soul	organs and systems of elimination and reproduction
Solar plexus	digestive system, liver, pancreas
Heart	heart, thymus, circulatory system
Throat	thyroid, lungs, respiratory system
Third eye	pituitary and portions of the brain
Crown	pineal, cerebral cortex, nervous system

MY PERSONAL PRAYER FOR HEALING

During my treatment for cancer I prayed each day to the angels and masters of healing. I formulated my prayer according to my own beliefs and understanding of my spiritual path. It includes specific tools and dispensations for healing. I found it to be very comforting and healing. As I prayed for myself, I also prayed for all who were burdened by cancer around the world.

You are welcome to use this prayer or to include portions of it in your own personal spiritual practice.

A Prayer for Healing

In the name I AM THAT I AM,[*] in the name of the Christ, I call to the legions of angels of divine healing and to Hilarion, the master of healing, to walk hand in hand with me this day and roll back the tidal wave that threatens the shore of my God-free being.[†]

I call for a wall of fire about me and the violet flame as the fire in the midst[‡] to seal my aura and my four lower bodies in the light and protection of God.

---

[*] Exod. 3:14.
[†] Saint Hilarion is known for turning back a tidal wave threatening to engulf the town where he lived.
[‡] Zech. 2:5.

I call forth the golden armor of Kuan Yin: the helmet, breastplate, back plate, shield, and buckler* and her circle and sword of mercy's flame. I ask for this armor of protection to be concealed within her cloak of invisibility, so that any weaknesses or vulnerable areas within my being and world are camouflaged from the prying eyes of the dark forces. Let not any point of vulnerability be used by the dark forces to derail or distract me from my mission and path.

I call to the saints both East and West for your momentum of the flame of the Prince of Peace, the purple and gold tinged with the ruby ray, drawn forth from the Elohim of Peace. I ask for the undulating rainbow rays, under the trained and expert beings of light who command them, to come now into my body and dissolve the cancer in my breast and anywhere else it is found. May these rainbow rays of God remove the cause and core of this condition. I call for the X-rays of God to "x" out any misuse of life and the life force in my body temple.

I call to God the Father to release into my desire body his desiring for my soul, to release into my heart chakra his love and his will, so that I might experience in my body temple the true presence, divine knowledge, and wisdom of the Father. I ask for my heart and being to be drawn into the mighty figure-eight flow with my Father's heart. For I know that when it comes to the difficult initiations of the secret rays, there is only one answer: be one with the Father, experience his heart, and do not doubt when you feel that presence and that answer.

Beloved Elohim of Peace, place your great sun disc over my solar plexus. I call in the name of the Christ for my aura, chakras and being to be fortified in God-control by God-mastery of the solar plexus. I call to Saint Bonaventure for the mastery of the solar plexus as one of the greatest assistances I can ever have and the key to my victory.

Be still, and know that I AM God.† (3x)

I call for the rivers of living water to flow from my belly, and I now

---

* Eph. 6:11–17.
† Ps. 46:10.

see my solar plexus as a fountain of peace, power, and plenty.* I cast out the forces of doubt and fear, and I call for an ovoid of fire to seal me.

I contemplate now the love of God and the presence of all the angels and masters of light. This calm and peaceful knowing of their presence does now dissolve all anxiety and fear, all self-doubt. I remain centered in the flame so that all those things can go quickly into the flame and so that the moment of pain will only be the moment of the passage of these things out of my aura.

I call to the masters of the seven rays to take me to the retreats of light in the heaven-world while my body sleeps at night. I ask them to explain to me specifically what are my karmic circumstances and my personality patterns and my habits of the human psyche so that I may no longer be bound by these limiting matrices. Let them be replaced by the pattern of my Christhood. I break the old cups, I dash the old bottles, and I pour the new wine into new wineskins.

Beloved Mother Mary and Archangel Raphael, place your healing thoughtform over my heart, mind, and solar plexus twenty-four hours a day. Beloved seraphim of God, place your fiery presence around me twenty-four hours a day to dissolve all impurities, all that is less than the Christ light, and all traces of cancer.

In the name of the Christ, I invoke the sealing of the mind with the emerald-teal ray. I invoke the dispensation from cosmic councils of the guardian action of the mind. I ask the special legions of angels to come forth for the sealing of my mental body and mind in a forcefield of brilliant, emerald-teal light. Let this light form a fine line of energy around the chakras of the crown, third eye, and head area, protecting and sealing my consciousness.

I claim the mantle of Bonaventure and the sphere of light from his causal body that I may access it any hour of the day or night. I call in the name of the Divine Mother for the resurrection flame and the resurrection spiral to pass through me twenty-four hours a day by the caduceus action, as Above, so below. I am sealed and comforted, close

---

*John 7:38.

and warm in the white wool mantle of the saints.
Let God's holy will be done. (3x)
Peace, be still, and know that I AM God. (3x)

Here is a prayer I gave many times while on my healing journey. I used it as a mantra and a meditation, visualizing the light penetrating my mind, my emotions, and my body, healing all levels of my being.

I AM Light

I AM Light, glowing Light,
Radiating Light, intensified Light.
God consumes my darkness,
Transmuting it into Light.

This day I AM a focus of the Central Sun.
Flowing through me is a crystal river,
A living fountain of Light
That can never be qualified
By human thought and feeling.
I AM an outpost of the divine.
Such darkness as has used me is swallowed up
By the mighty river of Light which I AM!

I AM, I AM, I AM Light.
I live, I live, I live in Light.
I AM Light's fullest dimension;
I AM Light's purest intention.
I AM Light, Light, Light
Flooding the world everywhere I move,
Blessing, strengthening, and conveying
The purpose of the kingdom of heaven.[1]

NOTES

Prologue

1. Luke 4:23.

Chapter 5

1. Patrick Quillin, "The Breast Cancer/Nutrition Connection," *Cancer Update* (Arlington Heights, Ill.: Cancer Treatment Centers of America), Summer 1999, p. 2.

Chapter 6

1. Bernie Siegel, *Love, Medicine and Miracles* (New York: Harper & Row, 1986), p. 25.
2. Dr. Isadore Rosenfeld, *Second Opinion: Your Comprehensive Guide to Treatment Alternatives,* quoted in Peggy Huddleston, *Prepare for Surgery, Heal Faster: A Guide of Mind-Body Techniques* (Cambridge, Mass.: Angel River Press, 1996), pp. 20–21.
3. Spiegel, D., et al. "Effects of Psychosocial Treatment on Survival of Patients with Metastatic Breast Cancer," *Lancet* (1989); ii: 888–91. Quoted in Steve Austin, N.D., and Cathy Hitchcock, M.S.W., *Breast Cancer: What You Should Know (But May Not Be Told) about Prevention, Diagnosis, and Treatment* (Rocklin, Calif.: Prima Publishing, 1994).

Chapter 7

1. Peggy Huddleston, *Prepare for Surgery, Heal Faster: A Guide of Mind-Body Techniques* (Cambridge, Mass.: Angel River Press, 1996), p. 2.
2. Siegel, *Love, Medicine and Miracles,* pp. 49, 47.
3. For information about the body elemental, see Mark L. Prophet and Elizabeth Clare Prophet, *The Path of the Higher Self* (Gardiner, Mont.: Summit University Press, 2003), pp. 380–86.
4. A good source of information about herbal remedies to assist in recovery from breast-cancer surgery is Susan S. Weed, *Breast Cancer? Breast Health! The Wise Woman Way* (Woodstock, N.Y.: Ash Tree Pub., 1996).

Chapter 8

1. Michael Castleman, *Blended Medicine: The Best Choices in Healing* (Emmaus, Pa.: Rodale Press, 2000), p. 6.
2. For more about cranberry juice and other natural remedies for urinary-tract infection, see Castleman, *Blended Medicine.*

Chapter 9

1. Cancer Treatment Centers of America website: www.cancercenter.com, *s.v.* Nutrition Support.
2. Patrick Quillin, "The Breast Cancer/Nutrition Connection," *Cancer Update*, Summer 1999, p. 2.
3. Ibid.
4. Bob Arnot, *The Breast Cancer Prevention Diet* (Boston: Little, Brown, and Company, 1998), pp. 67–91.
5. Quillin, "The Breast Cancer/Nutrition Connection."
6. Arnot, *The Breast Cancer Prevention Diet*, p. 19.
7. Michael Murray et al., *How to Prevent and Treat Cancer with Natural Medicine* (New York: Riverhead Books, 2002), p. 84.
8. Carter, J. P., et al. "Hypothesis: dietary management may improve survival from nutritionally linked cancers based on analysis of representative cases," *J Am Coll Nutr* 1993;12:209–26, quoted in Austin and Hitchcock, *Breast Cancer: What You Should Know (But May Not Be Told) About Prevention, Diagnosis, and Treatment*, pp. 137–38.
9. For a detailed discussion on the links between overweight and breast cancer, see Austin and Hitchcock, *Breast Cancer: What You Should Know (But May Not Be Told) About Prevention, Diagnosis, and Treatment*, pp. 240–44. For links to other forms of cancer, see National Cancer Institute FactSheet "Obesity and Cancer: Questions and Answers," available online at http://www.cancer.gov/cancertopics/factsheet/Risk/obesity
10. Thomas P. Lenz, "Vitamin D Supplementation and Cancer Prevention," *American Journal of Lifestyle Medicine*, vol. 3, no. 5, pp. 365–368; Stefan Pilz et.al., "Epidemiology of Vitamin D Insufficiency and Cancer Mortality," *Anticancer Research*, vol. 29, no. 9, pp. 3699–3704.

Chapter 10

1. Linn Goldberg and Diane L. Elliot, eds., *Exercise for Prevention and Treatment of Illness* (Philadelphia: F. A. Davis, 1994), p. vii. Quoted in Sala Horowitz, "Using the Body to Heal the Body," *Alternative & Complementary Therapies*, June 1998.
2. Patrick Quillin, "The Breast Cancer/Nutrition Connection," *Cancer Update*, Summer 1999, p. 2.
3. Murray, *How to Prevent and Treat Cancer with Natural Medicine*, pp. 15, 113–15.
4. Patrick Quillin, *Beating Cancer with Nutrition* (Tulsa, Okla.: Nutrition Times Press, 1998), pp. 20–21.
5. S. Blazickova, J. Rovensky, J. Koska, M. Vigas, "Effect of Hyperthermic Water Bath on Parameters of Cellular Immunity," *Int. J. Clin. Pharmacol. Res.*, 2000;20:41–46, quoted in Murray, *How to Prevent and Treat Cancer with Natural*

Medicine, p. 199; Quillin, *Beating Cancer with Nutrition,* p. 35.

6. Sandy Boucher, "Yoga for Cancer," *Yoga Journal,* May/June 1999.

7. Mark L. Prophet and Elizabeth Clare Prophet, *The Lost Teachings of Jesus* I (Gardiner, Mont.: Summit University Press, 1994), ch. 7, "Vitality and Prana."

Chapter 11

1. David Bognar, *Cancer: Increasing Your Odds for Survival* (Alameda, Calif.: Hunter House Publishers, 1998), p. 78.

2. Ibid., p. 79.

3. Siegel, *Love, Medicine, and Miracles,* p. 129.

4. Sari Harrar and Sara Altshul O'Donnell, *The Woman's Book of Healing Herbs, Healing Tonics, Teas, Supplements, and Formulas* (Emmaus, Pa.: Rodale Press, 1999), p. 24.

5. For a discussion on the scientific evidence for the use of melatonin in cancer treatment, see Murray, *How to Prevent and Treat Cancer with Natural Medicine,* pp. 242–44.

6. Dianne C. Witter, "Can a Common Spice Be Used to Treat Cancer?" *OncoLog,* Vol. 52, No. 9, September 2007.

7. American Cancer Society, "Modified Citrus Pectin," accessed at http://www.cancer.org/Treatment/TreatmentsandSideEffects/ComplementaryandAlternativeMedicine/DietandNutrition/modified-citrus-pectin November 7, 2010; University of California at San Diego, Moores Cancer Center, "Modified Citrus Pectin," accessed at http://cancer.ucsd.edu/outreach/PublicEducation/CAMs/modifiedcitrus.asp November 7, 2010.

8. Mechtild Scheffer, *Bach Flower Therapy: Theory and Practice* (Rochester, Vt.: Healing Arts Press, 1988), p. 9.

9. Elizabeth Clare Prophet and Patricia R. Spadaro, *Your Seven Energy Centers* (Gardiner, Mont.: Summit University Press, 2000), p. 211.

10. Information on the properties and uses of the Bach Flower Remedies and the specific remedies mentioned here is drawn from *Bach Flower Essences for the Family* (London: Wigmore Publications Ltd., 1996), *The Bach Flower Remedies* (New Canaan, Conn.: Keats Pub., 1997), and Patricia Kaminski and Richard Katz, *Flower Essence Repertory* (Nevada City, Calif.: Flower Essence Society, 1996).

11. Edward Bach, "The Twelve Healers," in *The Bach Flower Remedies.*

12. *Bach Flower Essences for the Family,* p. 24.

13. Kaminski and Katz, *Flower Essence Repertory,* p. 399.

14. Ibid., p. 400.

15. Much of the information included here on essential oils is found in Gary Young, *Introduction to Young Living Essential Oils* (Payson, Ut.: Young Living Essential Oils, 2000).

16. Castleman, *Blended Medicine,* p. 175.

Chapter 12

1. Sydney Ross Singer and Soma Grissmaijer, *Dressed to Kill: The Link between Breast Cancer and Bras* (Garden City Park, N.Y.: Avery Publishing Group, 1995).

Chapter 13

1. Joan Borysenko, *Minding the Body, Mending the Mind* (New York: Bantam Books, 1988), p. 26.
2. Siegel, *Love, Medicine and Miracles*, p. 3.
3. See Martin L. Rossman, *Healing Yourself: A Step-by-Step Program for Better Health through Imagery* (New York: Pocket Books, 1989), and Siegel, *Love, Medicine, and Miracles*, pp. 152–56. Dr. Rossman gives detailed explanations for the use of imagery for the healing of many different conditions. His book also includes many case studies of remarkable healings using these techniques.
4. For further information about the healing thoughtform, see Mark L. Prophet and Elizabeth Clare Prophet, *The Science of the Spoken Word* (Gardiner, Mont.: Summit University Press, 1991), pp. 144–48.
5. C. Norman Shealy, *Sacred Healing: The Curing Power of Energy and Spirituality* (Boston, Mass.: Element, 1999), p. 125.
6. Ibid., p. 124.
7. Andrew Weil, *Natural Health, Natural Medicine: A Comprehensive Manual for Wellness and Self-Care* (Boston: Houghton Mifflin, 1995), p. 188.
8. John Link, *The Breast Cancer Survival Manual: A Step-by-Step Guide for the Woman with Newly Diagnosed Breast Cancer* (New York: Henry Holt, 1998), p. 135.
9. Ibid.
10. Ibid., p. 189.
11. Lawrence LeShan, *Cancer as a Turning Point: A Handbook for People with Cancer, Their Families, and Health Professionals* (New York: Plume, 1994), p. xii.
12. Ibid., p. 24.
13. Ibid., p. 29.
14. Kuthumi, "Remember the Ancient Encounter," *Pearls of Wisdom* 28, no. 9, (1985). The Summit Lighthouse.
15. Louise L. Hay, *Heal Your Body: The Mental Causes for Physical Illness and the Metaphysical Way to Overcome Them* (Carlsbad, Calif.: Hay House, 1988), pp. 21, 22.
16. Ibid.
17. Bernie S. Siegel, *Peace, Love, and Healing: Bodymind Communication and the Path to Self-Healing: An Exploration* (New York: Harper & Row, 1989), p. 27.
18. Ibid., pp. 28, 162.
19. Siegel, *Love, Medicine, and Miracles*, p. 4.
20. Prov. 23:7.

21. Robert L. Van de Castle, *Our Dreaming Mind: A Sweeping Exploration of the Role That Dreams Have Played in Politics, Art, Religion, and Psychology, from Ancient Civilizations to the Present Day* (New York: Ballantine Books, 1995), pp. 364–65.

22. Ibid., p. 369.

23. Siegel, *Love, Medicine, and Miracles*, p. 114.

24. LeShan, *Cancer as a Turning Point*, p. 41.

25. Castleman, *Blended Medicine*, p. 79.

26. Mary Laney, "The Healing Power of Harps," *Chicago Tribune*, Sunday, December 11, 1994.

27. Siegel, *Peace, Love and Healing*, pp. 46–50.

Chapter 14

1. Siegel, *Peace, Love and Healing*, p. 2.

2. Larry Dossey, *Healing Words: The Power of Prayer and the Practice of Medicine* (San Francisco: HarperSanFrancisco, 1993), p. xviii.

3. Larry Dossey, *Prayer Is Good Medicine: How to Reap the Healing Benefits of Prayer* (San Francisco: HarperSanFrancisco, 1996), pp. 1–2.

4. Dossey, *Healing Words*, p. 180.

5. Paramahansa Yogananda, *Man's Eternal Quest* (Los Angeles: Self-Realization Fellow-ship, 1975), p. 43.

6. Elizabeth Clare Prophet, *The Creative Power of Sound* (Gardiner, Mont.: Summit University Press, 1998), pp. 49–53.

7. Borysenko, *Minding the Body, Mending the Mind*, p. 50.

8. This exercise is adapted from Elizabeth Clare Prophet, *Pearls of Wisdom* 30, no. 7 (1987).

9. Exod. 28:17–21, 39:10–14; Rev. 21:19–20.

10. The description of the properties of the amethyst is adapted from a lecture by Elizabeth Clare Prophet, 18 October 1987.

11. Melody, *Love Is in the Earth: A Kaleidoscope of Crystals* (Wheat Ridge, Col.: Earth-Love Publishing House, 1995), pp. 341–42.

12. Isa. 66:24.

13. Melody, *Love Is in the Earth*, p. 573.

14. Siegel, *Love, Medicine, and Miracles*, p. 29.

Chapter 15

1. Siegel, *Love, Medicine, and Miracles*, p. 133.

Chapter 16

1. El Morya, "Purity of Heart," *Pearls of Wisdom* 29, no. 80 (1986). El Morya,

"Job, the Chela of God," in *Keepers of the Flame Lesson 33* (Gardiner, Mont.: The Summit Lighthouse, 2001).

2. 1 John 4:4.

3. For a description of the initiations of the dark night, see Saint John of the Cross, "The Ascent of Mount Carmel" and "The Dark Night," in Kieran Kavanaugh and Otilio Rodriguez, trans., *The Collected Works of St. John of the Cross* (Washington, D.C.: ICS Publications, 1979), pp. 66–389; also commentary on the teachings of Saint John of the Cross in Elizabeth Clare Prophet, *Saint John of the Cross on the Living Flame of Love* (Gardiner, Mont.: Summit University, 1985), audio album.

4. For additional explanation of the dark night of the soul and the dark night of the Spirit, as well as the crucifixion as an initiation on the spiritual path, see Mark L. Prophet and Elizabeth Clare Prophet, *The Path of the Universal Christ* (Gardiner, Mont.: Summit University Press, 2003), pp. 167–213.

5. Matt. 27:46; Mark 15:34.

6. James 5:16.

7. A recently released biography of Edgar Cayce is Sidney D. Kirkpatrick, *Edgar Cayce: An American Prophet* (New York: Riverhead Books, 2000). See pp. 402–11 for an outline of the healing methods recommended by Cayce. Stories of Cayce's diagnoses may be found throughout the book.

8. Gladys Taylor McGarey, *The Physician within You: Medicine for the Millennium* (Deerfield Beach, Fla.: Health Communications, 1997), p. 37–39.

Chapter 17

1. Gal. 4:19.

2. John 1:19.

3. James 4:8.

4. Prophet, *Your Seven Energy Centers*, p. 65.

5. Robin Casarjian, *Forgiveness: A Bold Choice for a Peaceful Heart* (New York: Bantam Books, 1992), p. 236.

Appendix A

1. Information in this chart is from Elizabeth Clare Prophet and Patricia R. Spadaro, *Your Seven Energy Centers* (Gardiner, Mont.: Summit University Press, 2000).

Appendix B

1. Kuthumi and Djwal Kul, *The Human Aura* (Gardiner, Mont.: Summit University Press, 1982), p. 33.

RESOURCES

BOOKS:

Achterberg, Jeanne. *Imagery in Healing: Shamanism and Modern Medicine.* Boston: New Science Library, Shambhala, 1985.

Allegri, Renzo. *Padre Pio: Man of Hope.* Ann Arbor, Mich.: Servant Publications, 2000.

Arnot, Bob. *The Breast Cancer Prevention Diet: The Powerful Foods, Supplements, and Drugs That Can Save Your Life.* Boston, Mass.: Little, Brown, 1998.

Austin, Steve, and Cathy Hitchcock. *Breast Cancer: What You Should Know (But May Not Be Told) About Prevention, Diagnosis, and Treatment.* Rocklin, Calif.: Prima Pub., 1994.

Bach Flower Essences for the Family. London: Wigmore Publications Ltd., 1996.

The Bach Flower Remedies. New Canaan, Conn.: Keats Pub., 1997.

Barrick, Marilyn C. *Dreams: Exploring the Secrets of Your Soul.* Gardiner, Mont.: Summit University Press, 2001.

———. *Emotions: Transforming Anger, Fear and Pain.* Gardiner, Mont.: Summit University Press, 2002.

———. *Soul Reflections: Many Lives, Many Journeys.* Gardiner, Mont.: Summit University Press, 2003.

Benson, Herbert, with Miriam Z. Klipper. *The Relaxation Response.* New York: Wings Books, 1992.

Benson, Herbert, with Marg Stark. *Timeless Healing: The Power and Biology of Belief.* New York: Simon & Schuster, 1997.

Blofeld, John. *Bodhisattva of Compassion: The Mystical Tradition of Kuan Yin.* Boston: Shambhala Publications, Shambhala Dragon Editions, 1988.

Bognar, David. *Cancer: Increasing Your Odds for Survival: A Resource Guide for Integrating Mainstream, Alternative, and Complementary Therapies.* Alameda, Calif.: Hunter House Publishers, 1998.

Borysenko, Joan. *Guilt Is the Teacher, Love Is the Lesson.* New York: Warner Books, 1990.

Borysenko, Joan, and Miroslav Borysenko. *The Power of the Mind to Heal.*

Carson, Calif.: Hay House, 1994.

Borysenko, Joan, with Larry Rothstein. *Minding the Body, Mending the Mind.* New York: Bantam Books, 1988.

Burdine, Sally Astor. *Who Needs Hair ... The Flipside of Chemotherapy.* Bluewater Bay, Fla.: Saba Books, 2001.

Campbell, Don. *The Mozart Effect: Tapping the Power of Music to Heal the Body, Strengthen the Mind, and Unlock the Creative Spirit.* New York: Avon Books, 1997.

———. *Music and Miracles.* Wheaton, Ill.: Quest Books, 1992.

———, comp. *Music: Physician for Times to Come: An Anthology.* Wheaton, Ill.: Theosophical Pub. House, 1991.

Cancer Treatment Centers of America. *The Cancer Resource Guide: Dealing with the Cosmetic Side Effects of Your Treatment,* n.d.

Casarjian, Robin. *Forgiveness: A Bold Choice for a Peaceful Heart.* New York: Bantam Books, 1992.

Castleman, Michael. *Blended Medicine: How to Integrate the Best Mainstream and Alternative Remedies for Maximum Health and Healing.* Emmaus, Pa.: Rodale Books, 2002.

Clifford, Christine. *Not Now ... I'm Having a No Hair Day.* Duluth, Min.: Pfeifer-Hamilton Publishers, 1996.

Cousins, Norman. *Anatomy of an Illness as Perceived by the Patient: Reflections on Healing and Regeneration.* Boston: G. K. Hall, 1980.

Delaney, Gayle. *All About Dreams: Everything You Need to Know About Why We Have Them, What They Mean, and How to Put Them to Work for You.* San Francisco: HarperSanFrancisco, 1998.

Diamond, W. John, and W. Lee Cowden with Burton Goldberg. *An Alternative Medicine Definitive Guide to Cancer.* Tiburon, Calif.: Future Medicine Pub., 1997.

Dossey, Larry. *Be Careful What You Pray For ... You Just Might Get It: What We Can Do About the Unintentional Effects of Our Thoughts, Prayers, and Wishes.* San Francisco: HarperSanFrancisco, 1997.

———. *Healing Words: The Power of Prayer and the Practice of Medicine.* San Francisco: HarperSanFrancisco, 1993.

———. *Prayer is Good Medicine: How to Reap the Healing Benefits of Prayer.* San Francisco: HarperSanFrancisco, 1996.

Epstein, Samuel S., and David Steinman, with Suzanne LeVert. *The Breast Cancer Prevention Program.* New York: Macmillan, 1997.

Erasmus, Udo. *Fats That Heal, Fats That Kill: The Complete Guide to Fats, Oils, Cholesterol, and Human Health.* Burnaby, BC, Canada: Alive Books, 1993.

Faraday, Ann. *Dream Power.* New York: Coward, McCann & Geoghegan, 1972.

Harpham, Wendy Schlessel. *After Cancer: A Guide to Your New Life.* New York: HarperPerennial, 1995.

Harrar, Sari and Sara Altshul O'Donnell. *The Woman's Book of Healing Herbs: Healing Tonics, Teas, Supplements, and Formulas.* Emmaus, Pa.: Rodale Press, 1999.

Hay, Louise L. *Heal Your Body: The Mental Causes for Physical Illness and the Metaphysical Way to Overcome Them.* Santa Monica, Calif.: Hay House, 1988.

———. *You Can Heal Your Life.* Santa Monica, Calif.: Hay House, 1987.

Hersh, Stephen. *Beyond Miracles: Living with Cancer: Inspirational and Practical Advice for Patients and Their Families.* Lincolnwood, Ill.: Contemporary Books, 1998.

Hirshaut, Yashar, and Peter Pressman. *Breast Cancer: The Complete Guide.* New York: Bantam Books, 1992.

Huddleston, Peggy. *Prepare for Surgery, Heal Faster.* Cambridge, Mass.: Angel River Press, 1996. Companion audiocassette is also available.

Jahnke, Roger. *The Healer Within: The Four Essential Self-Care Methods for Creating Optimal Health: Movement, Massage, Meditation, and Breathing.* San Francisco, Calif.: HarperSanFrancisco, 1997.

Saint John of the Cross. "The Ascent of Mount Carmel" and "The Dark Night," in *The Collected Works of St. John of the Cross.* trans. Kieran Kavanaugh and Otilio Rodriguez. Washington, D.C.: ICS Publications, 1979.

Kalter, Suzy. *Looking Up: The Complete Guide to Looking and Feeling Good for the*

Recovering Cancer Patient. New York: McGraw-Hill, 1987.

Kaminski, Patricia, and Richard Katz. *Flower Essence Repertory.* Nevada City, Calif.: Flower Essence Society, 1996.

King, Dean, Jessica King and Jonathan Pearlroth. *Cancer Combat: Cancer Survivors Share Their Guerilla Tactics to Help You Win the Fight of Your Life.* New York: Bantam Books, 1998.

Kohler, Jean Charles, and Mary Alice Kohler. *Healing Miracles from Macrobiotics: A Diet for All Diseases.* West Nyack, N.Y.: Parker Pub. Co., 1979.

Kushi, Michio, with Alex Jack. *The Cancer Prevention Diet: Michio Kushi's Macrobiotic Blueprint for the Prevention and Relief of Disease.* New York: St. Martin's Press, 1994.

LaTour, Kathy. *The Breast Cancer Companion: From Diagnosis through Treatment to Recovery: Everything You Need to Know for Every Step along the Way.* New York: Avon Books, 1993.

LeShan, Lawrence. *Cancer as a Turning Point: A Handbook for People with Cancer, Their Families, and Health Professionals.* New York: Plume, 1994.

———. *How to Meditate: A Guide to Self-Discovery.* Boston: Little, Brown, 1974.

Link, John S. *The Breast Cancer Survival Manual: A Step-by-Step Guide for the Woman with Newly Diagnosed Breast Cancer.* New York: Henry Holt, 1998.

Love, Susan M., with Karen Lindsey. *Dr. Susan Love's Breast Book.* Reading, Mass.: Addison-Wesley, 1995.

McGarey, Gladys Taylor, with Jess Stearn. *The Physician within You: Medicine for the Millennium.* Deerfield Beach, Fla.: Health Communications, 1997.

Mauney, Thad. *Preventing and Reversing Breast Cancer Naturally—A Science-Based Nutritional Approach to Protecting Yourself From Breast and Other Cancers.* 2008.

Melody. *Love Is in the Earth: A Kaleidoscope of Crystals.* Wheat Ridge, Col.: Earth-Love Publishing House, 1995.

Michnovicz, Jon J. *How to Reduce Your Risk of Breast Cancer.* New York: Warner Books, 1994.

Morris, Virginia B., and Sophie Forrester. *A Patient's Guide to Cancer Care.* New York: Lightbulb Press, 2003.

Moss, Ralph W. *Herbs against Cancer: History and Controversy*. Brooklyn, N.Y.: Equinox Press, 1998.

Muramoto, Noboru B. *Natural Immunity: Insights on Diet and AIDS*. Oroville, Calif.: George Ohsawa Macrobiotic Foundation, 1988.

Murray, Michael T., Tim Birdsall, Joseph E. Pizzorno, and Paul Reilly. *How to Prevent and Treat Cancer with Natural Medicine*. New York: Riverhead Books, 2003.

Pelton, Ross, Taffy Clarke Pelton, and Vinton C. Vint. *How to Prevent Breast Cancer: A Lifestyle Guide for the Prevention of Breast Cancer and Its Recurrence—With an Investigation of Critical Risk Factors*. New York: Simon & Schuster, 1995.

Prophet, Elizabeth Clare. *Access the Power of Your Higher Self*. Gardiner, Mont.: Summit University Press, 1997.

——. *The Creative Power of Sound*. Gardiner, Mont.: Summit University Press, 1998.

——. *How to Work with Angels*. Gardiner, Mont.: Summit University Press, 1998.

Prophet, Elizabeth Clare, and Patricia Spadaro. *Your Seven Energy Centers*. Gardiner, Mont.: Summit University Press, 2000.

Prophet, Mark L., and Elizabeth Clare Prophet. *The Path of the Universal Christ*. Gardiner, Mont.: Summit University Press, 2003.

——. *The Science of the Spoken Word*. Gardiner, Mont.: Summit University Press, 1991.

——. *Understanding Yourself: A Spiritual Approach to Self-Discovery and Soul-Awareness*. Gardiner, Mont.: Summit University Press, 1999.

——. *The Human Aura, by Kuthumi and Djwal Kul*. Gardiner, Mont.: Summit University Press, 1996.

Quillin, Patrick. *Healing Nutrients: The People's Guide to Using Common Nutrients That Will Help You Feel Better than You Ever Thought Possible*. New York: Vintage Books, 1989.

——. *Adjuvant Nutrition in Cancer Treatment*. Arlington Heights, Ill.: Cancer Treatment Research Foundation, 1994.

Quillin, Patrick, with Noreen Quillin. *Beating Cancer with Nutrition: Clinically*

Proven and Easy-to-Follow Strategies to Dramatically Improve Quality and Quantity of Life and Chances for a Complete Remission. Tulsa, Okla.: Nutrition Times Press, 1998.

Randolph, Theron G., and Ralph W. Moss. *An Alternative Approach to Allergies: The New Field of Clinical Ecology Unravels the Environmental Causes of Mental and Physical Ills.* New York: Lippincott & Crowell, 1980.

Read, Cathy. *Preventing Breast Cancer: The Politics of an Epidemic.* Hammersmith, London; San Francisco, Calif.: Pandora, 1995.

Rossman, Martin L. *Healing Yourself: A Step-by-Step Program for Better Health through Imagery.* New York: Walker, 1987.

Runowicz, Carolyn D., and Donna Haupt. *To Be Alive: A Woman's Guide to a Full Life after Cancer.* New York: Holt, 1995.

Scheffer, Mechthild. *Bach Flower Therapy: Theory and Practice.* Rochester, Vt.: Healing Arts Press, 1986.

Shealy, C. Norman. *Sacred Healing: The Curing Power of Energy and Spirituality.* Boston, Mass.: Element, 1999.

Sheikh, Anees A., Katharina Sheikh, eds. *Healing East and West: Ancient Wisdom and Modern Psychology.* New York: Wiley, 1996.

Siegel, Bernie S. *How to Live between Office Visits: A Guide to Life, Love, and Health.* New York: HarperCollins, 1993.

———. *Love, Medicine, and Miracles: Lessons Learned about Self-Healing from a Surgeon's Experience with Exceptional Patients.* New York: HarperPerennial, 1990.

———. *Peace, Love, and Healing: Bodymind Communication and the Path to Self-Healing: An Exploration.* New York: Harper & Row, 1989.

Simonton, O. Carl, Stephanie Matthews-Simonton and James Creighton. *Getting Well Again: A Step-by-Step Self-Help Guide to Overcoming Cancer for Patients and Their Families.* Los Angeles: J. P. Tarcher, 1978.

Smith, Ed. *Therapeutic Herb Manual: A Guide to the Safe and Effective Use of Liquid Herbal Extracts.* Williams, Ore.: Ed Smith, 1999.

Spiller, Gene, and Bonnie Bruce. *Cancer Survivor's Nutrition and Health Guide: Eating Well and Getting Better During and After Cancer Treatment.* Rocklin, Calif.: Prima Pub., 1997.

Stumm, Dianna. *Recovering from Breast Surgery: Exercises to Strengthen Your Body and Relieve Pain.* Alameda, Calif.: Hunter House, 1995.

Swirsky, Joan, and Barbara Balaban. *The Breast Cancer Handbook: Taking Control after You've Found a Lump: A Step-by-Step Guide.* New York: HarperPerennial, 1994.

Tame, David. *The Secret Power of Music.* New York: Destiny Books, 1984.

Van de Castle, Robert L. *Our Dreaming Mind: A Sweeping Exploration of the Role That Dreams Have Played in Politics, Art, Religion, and Psychology, from Ancient Civilizations to the Present Day.* New York: Ballantine Books, 1995.

Vithoulkas, George. *The Science of Homeopathy.* New York: Grove Press, 1980.

Weed, Susan S. *Breast Cancer? Breast Health! The Wise Woman Way.* Woodstock, N.Y.: Ash Tree Pub., 1996.

Weil, Andrew. *Natural Health, Natural Medicine: A Comprehensive Manual for Wellness and Self-Care.* Boston: Houghton Mifflin, 1995.

Weiss, Marisa, and Ellen Weiss. *Living Beyond Breast Cancer: A Survivor's Guide for When Treatment Ends and the Rest of Your Life Begins.* New York: Times Books, 1998.

Yalof, Ina, ed. *Straight from the Heart: Letters of Hope and Inspiration from Survivors of Breast Cancer.* New York: Kensington Books, 1996.

Young, D. Gary. *An Introduction to Young Living Essential Oils.* Payson, Ut.: Young Living Essential Oils, 2000.

AUDIO RECORDINGS:

Campbell, Don. *Healing with Great Music.* Louisville, Col.: Sounds True, 1998.

———. *The Mozart Effect.* Grand Haven, Mich.: Brilliance Corp., 1997.

Fulton, Dorothy Lee. *Five Dhyani Buddhas.* Emigrant, Mont.: Cosmic Portals, n.d.

———. *Music of the Spheres.* Emigrant, Mont.: Cosmic Portals, n.d.

Hearts of Space. *Sacred Treasures: Choral Masterworks from Russia.* Sausalito, Calif.: Hearts of Space, 1998.

Huddleston, Peggy. *Prepare for Surgery, Heal Faster: Relaxation/Healing Audiotape.* Angel River Press, 1996. Companion audiocassette to the book of the same title.

Prophet, Elizabeth Clare. *Kuan Yin's Crystal Rosary: Devotions to the Divine Mother East and West*. Gardiner, Mont.: The Summit Lighthouse, 1988.

———. *Saint John of the Cross on the Living Flame of Love*. Gardiner, Mont.: Summit University, 1985.

———. *Spiritual Techniques to Heal Body, Mind, and Soul*. Gardiner, Mont.: The Summit Lighthouse, 1999.

Siegel, Bernie S. *Healing Meditations: Enhance Your Immune System and Find the Key to Good Health*. Carlsbad, Calif.: Hay House Audio, 2000.

Weil, Andrew. *Sound Body, Sound Mind: Music for Healing*. New York: Tommy Boy Music, 1998.

OTHER RESOURCES:

American Academy of Environmental Medicine
7701 East Kellogg, Suite 625, Wichita, KS, 67207
(316) 684-5500
www.aaem.org

American Cancer Society
1-800-ACS-2345
www.cancer.org

Cancer Treatment Centers of America
3150 Salt Creek Lane, Suite 118, Arlington Heights, IL, 60005
1-800-615-3055
www.cancercenter.com

ECaP (Exceptional Cancer Patients)
522 Jackson Park Drive, Meadville, PA, 16335
(814) 337-8192
www.ecap-online.org

The Summit Lighthouse
63 Summit Way
Gardiner, MT 59030-9314
(406) 848-9200
www.tsl.org

www.journeythroughcancer.org
Web site with much of the content of this book

Special thanks to Summit University Press for permission to include the following material: "I AM Light" © 1982; "Forgiveness" decree © 1962; Chart of Your Divine Self © 1977; Kuan Yin image © 1983; seven chakras image © 1994; Virgin of the Globe © 1992. For more information, contact Summit University Press®, 63 Summit Way, Gardiner, Montana 59030-9314. Tel. (406) 848-9500, E-mail: tslinfo@TSL.org. Web site: www.TSL.org.

CPSIA information can be obtained at www.ICGtesting.com
Printed in the USA
BVOW011316080412

287112BV00004B/8/P